NEURO-ONCOLOGY

DEVELOPMENTS IN ONCOLOGY

VOLUME 3

Previously published in this series:

1. F.J. Cleton and J.W.I.M. Simons, eds. Genetic Origins of Tumor Cells
   ISBN 90-247-2272-1
2. J. Aisner and P. Chang, eds. Cancer Treatment Research
   ISBN 90-247-2358-2

Series: ISBN 90-247-2338-8

NEURO-ONCOLOGY
Clinical and Experimental Aspects

Proceedings of the International Symposium on Neuro-Oncology,
Noordwijkerhout, The Netherlands, October 25–27, 1979

edited by

B.W. ONGERBOER DE VISSER

Municipal Hospital Slotervaart, and
The Netherlands Cancer Institute,
Amsterdam

D.A. BOSCH

University Hospital,
Groningen

W.M.H. VAN WOERKOM-EYKENBOOM

Rotterdamsch Radiotherapeutisch Instituut,
Rotterdam

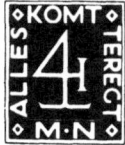

1980

SPRINGER-SCIENCE+BUSINESS MEDIA, B.V

ISBN 978-94-009-8921-4   ISBN 978-94-009-8919-1 (eBook)
DOI 10.1007/978-94-009-8919-1

TABLE OF CONTENTS

PREFACE

Neuro-oncology has been defined by J.B. Posner as a subspeciality of Neurology, which deals with the diagnosis and treatment of patients suffering from involvement of the nervous system by primary neoplasms, the effects of systemic cancer on the nervous system and with pain resulting from neoplastic involvement of either neural or non-neural structures.

The choice of neuro-oncology for this symposium organized by The Netherlands Society of Neurology emanated from Dr. L.J. Endtz, who is a delegate of the board, showed his continuous interest in the work of the committee, charged with its preparation. The symposium was actively supported by The Netherlands Society of Neurosurgeons and The Netherlands Society for Radiotherapy.

The purpose of this meeting was to bring together specialists of different medical disciplines to exchange and discuss information concerning the topics selected for this symposium. One of our aims was also to stress the importance of this rapidly developing subspeciality and to encourage practicing neurologists to take an active part in its development.

The large attendance and interested response to the presentations led us to believe that we met our goals and that the exchange of information in both the formal and informal sessions was valuable.

The editors hope that by publishing the formal proceedings to reach many more interested colleagues and to give some insight into the problems of neuro-oncology.

The Editors

LIST OF PARTICIPANTS

Ash, D., Radiotherapist, Cookridge Hospital, Leeds, England

Balhuizen, J.C., Pathologic Institute, Dordrecht, The Netherlands

Behrendt, H., Paediatrician, Emma Children's Hospital, Amsterdam,
The Netherlands

Bosch, D.A., Neurosurgeon, University Hospital, Groningen, The Netherlands

Bots, G.Th.A.M., Neuro-pathologist, University Hospital, Leiden, The Netherlands

Drenthe-Schonk, A.M., Haematologist, St. Radboud University Hospital, Nijmegen,
The Netherlands

Droog, R., Paediatrician, Emma Children's Hospital, Amsterdam, The Netherlands

Endtz, L.J. Neurologist, Municipal Hospitals, Leyenburg, The Hague, The Netherlands

Feltkamp, C.A., Electron-microscopist, The Netherlands Cancer Institute,
Amsterdam, The Netherlands

Feltkamp-Vroom, Th.M., Immuno-pathologist, Municipal Hospital Slotervaart,
Amsterdam, The Netherlands

Frederiks, J.A.M., Neurologist, St. Catharina Hospital, Eindhoven, The Netherlands

Graaf, Th.M., de, S.S.M., Paediatrician, University Hospital, Groningen,
The Netherlands

Greenberg, H.S., Neurologist, Memorial Sloan-Kettering Cancer Center, New York, USA

Goedhart, Z.D., Neurosurgeon, Municipal Hospital, Slotervaart, Amsterdam,
The Netherlands

Haanen, C., Haematologist, St. Radboud University Hospital, Nijmegen,
The Netherlands

Hansen, H.H., Internist, Finsen Institute, Copenhagen, Denmark

Hengefeld, J.W., Neurologist, Municipal Hospitals, Leyenburg, The Hague.
The Netherlands

Hildebrand, J., Neurologist, Institute Jules Bordet, Brussels, Belgium

Hirsch, F.R., Internist, Finsen Institute, Copenhagen, Denmark

Holleman, J., Internist, Rotterdamsch Radio-Therapeutisch Instituut, Rotterdam,
The Netherlands

Jonkers, A., Radiologist, University Hospital, Groningen, The Netherlands

Juel-Jensen, B.E., Epidemiologist, Radcliffe Infirmary, Oxford, England

Kamps, W.A., Paediatrician, University Hospital, Groningen, The Netherlands

Kendall, B.E., Neuro-radiologist, The National Hospital for Nervous Diseases,
.. London, England

Kingsley, D.P.E., Neuro-radiologist, The London Hospital, London, England

Mehta, D.M., Radiotherapist, University Hospital Groningen, The Netherlands

Meyer, E., Neurosurgeon, St. Radboud University Hospital, Nijmegen,
The Netherlands

Moffie, D., Neurologist, Municipal Hospital, Slotervaart, Amsterdam,
The Netherlands

Ongerboer de Visser, B.W., Neurologist, Municipal Hospital Slotervaart and
The Clinical Department of the Netherlands Cancer Institute, Amsterdam,
The Netherlands

Paulson, O.B., Neurologist, Righshospitalet, Copenhagen, Denmark

Posner, J.B., Neurologist, Memorial Sloan-Kettering Cancer Center, New York, USA

Postma, A., Paediatrician, University Hospital, Groningen, The Netherlands

Price, R.A., Pathologist, St. Jude Children's Research Hospital, Memphis,
Tennessee, USA

Rossum, J. van, Neurologist, University Hospital, Leiden, The Netherlands

Sizoo, W., Haematologist, Rotterdamsch Radio-Therapeutisch Instituut, Rotterdam,
The Netherlands

Somers, R., Haematologist, Clinical Department of The Netherlands Cancer
Institute, Amsterdam, The Netherlands

Stefanko, S.Z., Neuro-pathologist, Dijkzigt University Hospital, Rotterdam,
The Netherlands

Swen, J.W.A., Neurologist, Municipal Hospitals Leyenburg, The Hague,
The Netherlands

Voûte, P.A., Paediatrician, Emma Children's Hospital, Amsterdam, The Netherlands

Webb, H.E., Neurologist, St. Thomas' Hospital, London, England

Willemze, R., Haematologist, University Hospital, Leiden, The Netherlands

van Woerkom-Eykenboom, W.M.H., Radiotherapist, Rotterdamsch Radio-
Therapeutisch Instituut, Rotterdam, The Netherlands

1. NEURO-ONCOLOGY: AN OVERVIEW

J.B. Posner

Good morning. My name is Jerome Posner and I am from Memorial Sloan-Kettering Cancer Center in New York City. It is a signal honor to be invited by the Netherlands Societies of Neurology, Neurosurgery and Radiotherapy to give the opening remarks to this Conference on Neuro-Oncology. I am particularly pleased that the societies have selected neuro-oncology as a topic because it gives recognition to a field that has come of age and indicates that neurologists, neurosurgeons and radiotherapists should develop and expand their interests in the area.

What do we mean by neuro-oncology? (Table 1)

TABLE 1: DEFINITION OF NEURO-ONCOLOGY.

1) Subspecialty of neurology
2) Deals with diagnosis and treatment of patients suffering from:
    a) primary central nervous system (CNS) neoplasms,
    b) neurological complications of systemic cancer,
    c) pain.

For purposes of my discussion this morning, by neuro-oncology I mean an area of study which deals with: 1) the diagnosis and treatment of patients suffering from primary CNS neoplasms (brain and spinal cord tumors); 2) neurological complications of systemic cancer (cancer which arises outside the nervous system and affects the nervous system secondarily), and 3) pain associated with cancer. New developments in the neurophysiology and neuropharmacology of pain make it particularly important for neurologically trained physicians with a sophisticated knowledge of neurophysiology and neuropharmacology to participate in the diagnosis and treatment of patients suffering from pain related to cancer.

Why should neurologists be interested in neuro-oncology? The reasons are several (Table 2). I will dwell primarily on the neurological complications of systemic cancer and detail some of the reasons which should prompt neurological interest:

Table 2: NEURO-ONCOLOGY: REASONS FOR ITS IMPORTANCE

1) Disorders are common.
2) Incidence is increasing.
3) Suffering and disability are major.
4) Diagnosis is difficult.
5) Treatment helps.
6) Problems are unique.
7) Brain and cancer are related.

The first reason is that neurological complications of systemic cancer are common. At a cancer hospital such as Memorial Sloan-Kettering, neurologists are asked to see approximately 15% of all admissions because of a significant neurological complication of their primary disease.

The second reason is that there is evidence that the incidence of neurological complications of systemic cancer is increasing, not only in cancer hospitals but also in general hospitals where patients with cancer are cared for.

The third reason is that suffering and disability in patients with systemic cancer and its neurological complications are major. Dementia, hemiplegia or incontinence are tragic symptoms even in a patient with widespread cancer. For example, an individual with widespread bone metastases from breast cancer may be able to function normally, but if the nervous system becomes involved, she may become bedridden and be unable to continue her job or care for her family.

Furthermore, the diagnosis of the cause of neurological disability in a patient known to have cancer is not always easy, and considerable neurological sophistication frequently is required in order to make a definitive diagnosis.

However, correct neurological diagnosis is important because treatment directed at the nervous system complication often helps. Individuals are not cured of cancer by treatment directed at the CNS, but such treatment in a patient suffering from a neurological complication of cancer may return that individual to a state in which he can function and where the quality of life is considerably improved. For example, the patient with widespread carcinoma of the breast who develops a metastatic brain tumor can become hemiplegic and demented. If one effectively treats the brain tumor, even though she still has widespread metastatic carcinoma of the breast, she may improve enough to return to work or be at home in fairly comfortable surroundings rather than in a hospital or nursing home.

When cancer involves the nervous system, there are problems which are unique to the nervous system and which do not occur when other organs are involved by cancer. For example, there is the problem of the blood-brain barrier, which will be discussed in more detail in this conference later on.

Finally, there are interesting and unusual relationships between systemic cancer and the brain which we do not understand but which are probably very important from a neurobiological viewpoint. A portion of this conference is related to paraneoplastic syndromes - those syndromes in which the cancer damages a part of the nervous system without actually contacting it. An understanding of the pathogenesis of those syndromes should help both neurologists and oncologists understand the biology not only of the nervous system but also of systemic cancer itself.

Let us consider each of these in turn. I said neurological complications of systemic cancer are common, and Table 3 is one example:

Table 3: CANCER INCIDENCE: 1977				
Category	New Cases	Deaths	Intracranial Disease	
			#	%
All cancers	690,000	385,000		
Breast	89,700	34,000	10,200	30
Lung	98,000	89,000	30,260	34
Melanoma	9,500	5,300	3,816	72
Lymphoma	21,900	15,700	2,512	16
Leukemia	21,300	15,000	3,450	23

On the left are Silverberg's 1977 predictions of the incidence of cancer in the United States (1). In 1977, there were 690,000 new cases of cancer and 385,000 deaths in our population of about 220 million. There are approximately 1,000 deaths from cancer a day in our country. The data on the right are from a study at Memorial of the incidence of intracranial metastases found at autopsy (2). If one extrapolates our figures to the national numbers, one calculates that in the United States approximately 68,000 patients a year die with intracranial metastases from their systemic cancer. Of those 68,000 patients, approximately 2/3 will have suffered significant neurological symptoms during life (3).

Not only are the numbers of intracranial metastases large, but the incidence appears to be increasing. Figure 1 is from an autopsy study carried out by Dr. Norman Chernik at our institution. He plotted the prevalence of intracranial, intracerebral and leptomeningeal metastases at our hospital from the years 1970 to 1977 (2).

FIGURE 1:

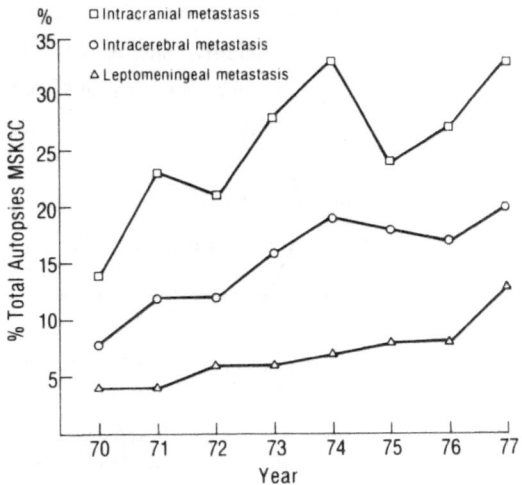

- The incidence and type of intracranial metastases encountered at autopsy at Memorial Sloan-Kettering Cancer Center in the years 1970 through 1977. Although there is wide variability in the overall incidence of particular types of metastasis from year to year, the trend has been a steadily increasing one, suggesting that intracranial metastases are indeed becoming a more common problem.

There has been a small but gradual increase in the incidence of each of these intracranial complications of metastatic cancer. Although there are difficulties in interpreting data from a single institution, more and more reports from other institutions have indicated an increasing incidence of intracranial lesions in patients suffering from systemic cancers of the ovary (4), small cell carcinoma of the lung (5) and even some sarcomas (6), all illnesses which sometimes respond to systemic chemotherapy. Because intracranial complications of systemic cancer appear to be increasing, I suspect the role of the neurologist, the neurosurgeon and the neuroradiotherapist will become greater and greater with the passage of time.

The diagnosis of neurological complications of systemic cancer is difficult and to a neurological audience I need not dwell on the difficulty of establishing a differential diagnosis in a patient suffering from suspected cancer and intracranial lesions. One example may suffice. A young woman was sent to us for RT because she had developed a progressive left hemiparesis over a 3-week period. There was a contrast-enhancing lesion in the CT scan of her right hemisphere (see Fig. 2). When her physician began corticosteroid therapy, she improved. There was no evidence of a primary tumor outside the nervous system, and her physician thought the lesion was too deep to biopsy, although under other circumstances we might have biopsied it.

FIGURE 2:

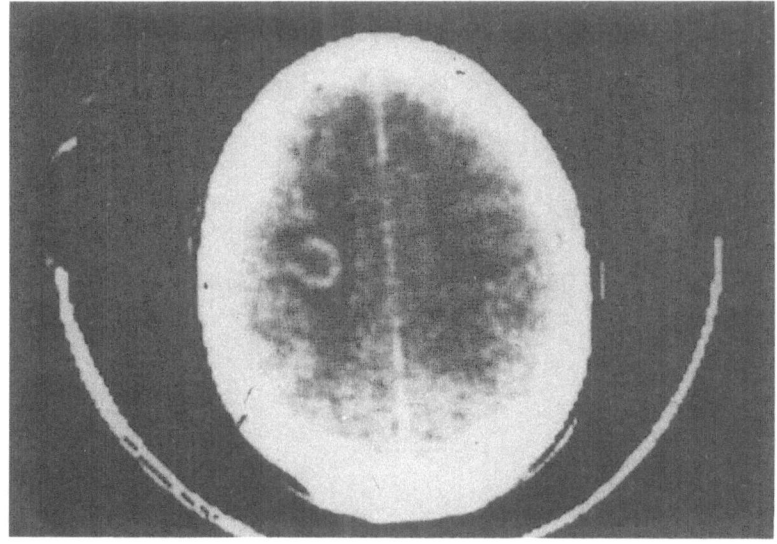

A careful neurological history, however, revealed that 3 years before she had had mild numbness and tingling on the entire right side of her body which had lasted 2 or 3 weeks and then disappeared spontaneously. We elected to follow this lesion rather than biopsy or radiate it; within a few months it disappeared. This was a couple of years ago, but all of you recognize this as a contrast-enhancing plaque of multiple sclerosis. Thus, diagnosis requires a physician who knows something not only aobut cancer but also about general neurology and the differential diagnosis of neurological disorders.

Treatment helps. Treatment vigorously directed at the nervous system can resolve neurological problems which arise either in the setting of systemic cancer or from cancer involving the nervous system primarily.

Figure 3A is the CT scan of a patient with a brain metastasis from an adenocarcinoma of the lung. She was hemiparetic. She received steroids and was treated with radiotherapy (3). She responded and became free of neurological symptoms. Figure 3B is a CT scan one year later.

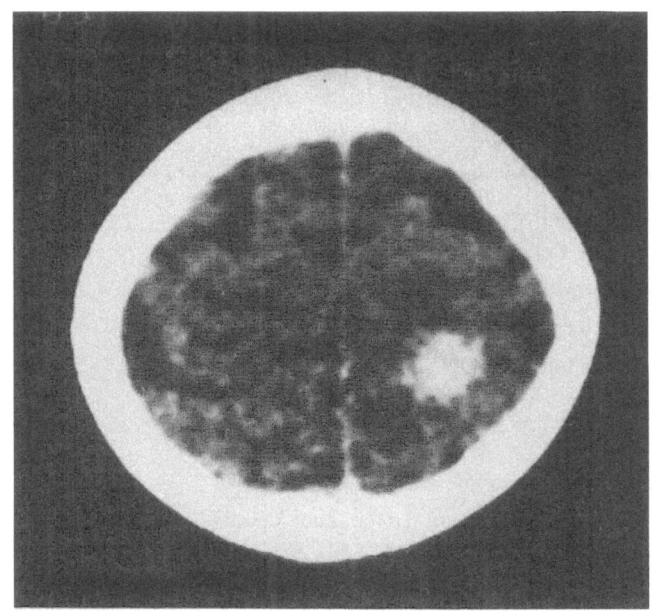

FIGURE 3A

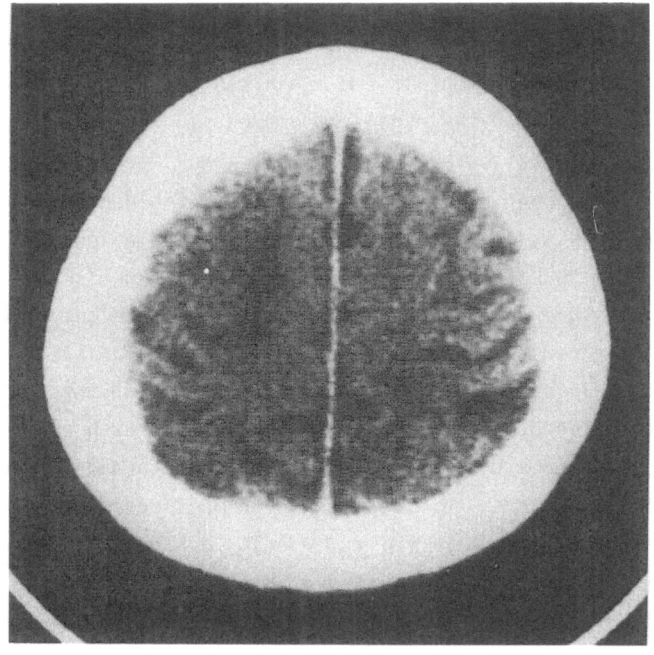

FIGURE 3B

Neurological complications of systemic cancer have unique aspects,
some of which are listed below (Table 4):

Table 4: UNIQUE ASPECTS OF BRAIN METASTASES.

1) The skull is a closed box.
   a) Tumor causes increased intracranial pressure.
   b) Tumor causes cerebral herniations.
2) Blood-brain barrier
   a) cerebral edema
   b) sanctuary for malignant cells
   c) exclusion of chemotherapeutic agents
   d) exclusion of toxic substances
3) No lymphatics
   a) poor drainage of edema
   b) ? poor drainage of toxic substances
4) The CNS does not regenerate.
   a) Neurologic disability, once established, may not reverse.

One unique aspect of the brain is that it and its surrounding
membranes are encased in a rigid box, the skull, which effectively
prevents expansion of the intracranial contents. Within the skull of
the brain are its blood supply and the cerebrospinal fluid. Increase
in the size of one compartment of the brain can only occur if there is
a decrease in the size of the other compartments. When new tissue,
such as a brain metastasis is introduced into the intracranial cavity,
the pressure within that cavity rises, quantity of blood and
cerebrospinal fluid is decreased, and there are herniations of
intracranial structures from one compartment to another. Rise in
intracranial pressure and the cerebral herniations lead to vascular
compromise and increase the symptoms of a brain metastasis.

The blood-brain barrier is another unique aspect of the central
nervous system. The blood-brain barrier breaks down as brain
metastases develops and this breakdown of the blood-brain barrier
leads to swelling which in turn increases cerebral pressure and causes
cerebral herniation. Furthermore, tumor cells behind an intact
blood-brain barrier may find a sanctuary which protects them from
chemotherapeutic agents delivered effective for tumor in the rest of
the body. This concept was based on the experience with acute

Table 5: NEUROLOGICAL COMPLICATIONS OF SYSTEMIC CANCER.

1) METASTATIC
        a) intracranial
        b) spinal
        c) meningeal
        d) peripheral nerve or plexus

2) NONMETASTATIC
        a) metabolic encephalopathy
        b) infections
        c) vascular disorders
        d) side effects of therapy
        e) "remote effects"

3) EITHER OR BOTH
        a) pain

If you stop to think about the ways in which cancer can affect the nervous system, there are essentially two: 1) Systemic cancer can metastasize to the nervous system, in which case the metastases can be subdivided anatomically for purposes of diagnosis and treatment. Today we are going to hear about intracranial metastases, spinal metastases and meningeal metastases and their treatment. We are not going to dwell on metastases of the peripheral nerves or plexuses, although they are becoming increasingly important, particularly those of the brachial plexus involved by cancer of both lung and breast. 2) There are nonmetastatic complications of systemic cancer, which include metabolic brain disease resulting from failure of systems outside the brain (e.g. liver failure, pulmonary failure), infections, vascular disorders, side effects of therapy and the paraneoplastic or remote effects of cancer on the nervous system. All of these are important both for management of the patient and for our understanding of disease processes. Let me give you a couple of examples:

Metabolic brain disease is important because oncologists frequently have difficulty distinguishing between neurological signs which develop because tumor has metastasized to the nervous system and neurological signs which develop because a systemic organ such as the liver is failing. When we came to look at the cause of death in patients whose intracranial metastases had been treated with RT, we discovered that, contrary to previous reports in the literature, patients died not of their brain disease, which responded to treatment, but of their systemic disease (3). The reason, I believe, that reports in the literature differ is because as systemic cancer begins to destroy the kidney or lungs, patients develop metabolic encephalopathy, leading the physician to conclude that they died of brain metastases rather than systemic disease. They are thus thought to be failures of RT to the brain when, in fact, the treatment to the brain has been successful.

A neurologist dealing with cancer also has to know about infections of the nervous system since they are common and differ from the infections one encounters in the general population. At our hospital the most common causes of meningitis are listeria and crypto-coccus, and the most common brain abscess is toxoplasma. Vascular disorders are likewise important. At our hospital the most common cause of stroke is nonbacterial thrombotic endocarditis with cerebral embolism. Arteriosclerotic strokes are relatively uncommon in our hospital, and Dr. Chernik has collected evidence that in fact the degree of cerebral arteriosclerosis in patients dying of cancer is considerably less in all age groups than is cerebral atherosclerosis in patients dying of some other illness (10). Side effects of therapy and remote effects of cancer on the nervous system are also important and will be discussed further in this conference.

I have intended this overview to point out some of the problems which face physicians dealing with neurological complications of systemic cancer and to set in perspective the interesting papers which we will hear during the next 2 days.

Thank you.

REFERENCES

1. Silverberg, E, Cancer statistics. Ca 27: 26, 1977
2. Posner, JB, and NL Chernik, Intracranial metastases from systemic cancer. Adv Neurol 19: 575, 1978
3. Cairncross, JG, J-H KIM and JB Posner, Radiation therapy of brain metastases. Ann Neurol (in press)
4. Mayer, RJ, RS Berkowitz, and CT Griffiths, Central nervous system involvement by ovarian carcinoma. Cancer 41: 776, 1970
5. Nugent, JL, et al, CNS metastases in small cell bronchogenic carcinoma. Increasing frequency and changing pattern with lengthening survival. Cancer 44: 1885, 1979
6. Gercovich, RG, MA Luna, and JA Gottlieb, Increased incidence of cerebral metastases in sarcoma patients with prolonged survival from chemotherapy. Report of cases of leiomyosarcoma and chondrosarcoma. Cancer 36: 1843, 1975
7. Vick, NA, JD Khandekar, and DD Bigner, Chemotherapy of brain tumors. Arch Neurol 34: 523, 1977
8. Blasberg, RG, et al, Metastatic brain tumors: local blood flow and capillary permeability. Neurology 29: 547, 1979
9. Cotzias, GC, and LC Tang, An adenylate cyclase of brain reflects propensity for breast cancer in mice. Science 197: 1094, 1977
10. Chernik, NL, RB Loewenson, JB Posner and JA Resch, Cerebral atherosclerosis and stroke in cancer patients. Neurol 28: 350, 1978

2. INVOLVEMENT OF THE NERVOUS SYSTEM IN METASTATIC DISEASE OF CHILDHOOD

D.P.E. Kingsley, B. Kendall

Metastatic tumours involving the central nervous system are considered to be rare in children (1); this is in marked contrast to adults in which metastases usually from a systemic primary tumour account for between 10 and 20% of intracranial tumours (2, 3, 4). In recent years improved therapy has prolonged life expectancy from many neoplasms which has increased the likelihood of eventual nervous system involvement by some tumours. Also the development of the effective and minimally invasive procedure of computed tomography has facilitated the detection of tumours in the nervous system. We considered that it would be of interest to assess the present incidence and the features, especially on computed tomograms, of involvement of the central nervous system by metastatic malignancy in children and have reviewed our material to this end.

METHODS

All cases of metastases diagnosed in the decade between 1969 and 1979 were obtained from the patient register at the Hospital for Sick Children, London and their records were evaluated for evidence of intracranial or spinal involvement. The patients were divided into five groups.

1. Intracranial metastases from a systemic primary tumour;
2. Cerebral metastases from a primary tumour of the nervous system;
3. Spinal metastases from a systemic primary tumour;
4. Spinal metastases associated with a primary tumour in the nervous system;
5. Systemic metastases from a primary tumour of the nervous system.

RESULTS

During the ten years up to 1979 we have been able to trace 238 cases
with proven metastases and of these there was involvement of the
intracranial central nervous system in 44, and of the spine in 17 cases.
In 52 of these, other systems were involved and in 9 central nervous
system spread was isolated.

GROUP 1

Cranial and cerebral metastases from a systemic primary

The origin of the primary tumour and the time between the diagnosis of
the primary and metastatic lesions of the 22 cases are shown in Table 1.
Of the 89 neuroblastomas which produced metastases, 15 (17%) caused
cranial involvement usually associated with extradural masses, which
occasionally appeared to extend through the dura. The metastases were
single in 7 and multiple in 8 cases; all but one involved the adjacent
bone (figure 1) and there was widening with erosions of the sutures in
7 cases (figure 2).

a 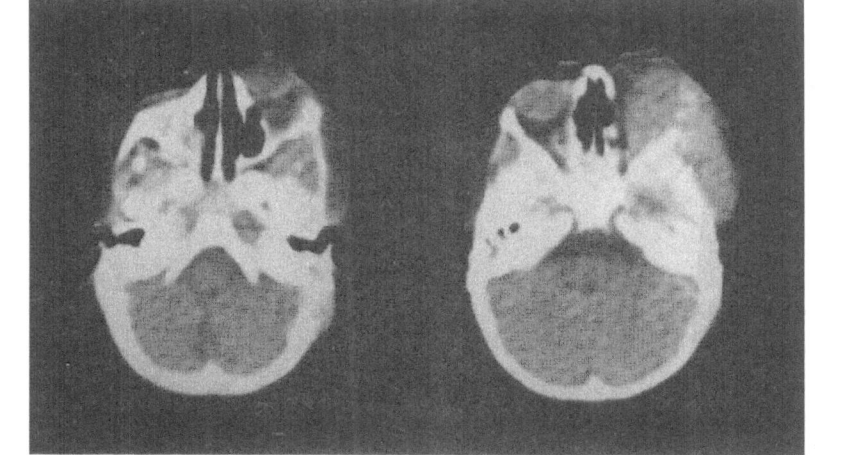 b

Figure 1: Neuroblastoma. CT adjacent sections through orbit and middle
fossa. There is destruction of the lateral wall of the right orbit
with a large continuous soft tissue mass within the orbital cavity and
temporal fossa. There is marked proptosis.

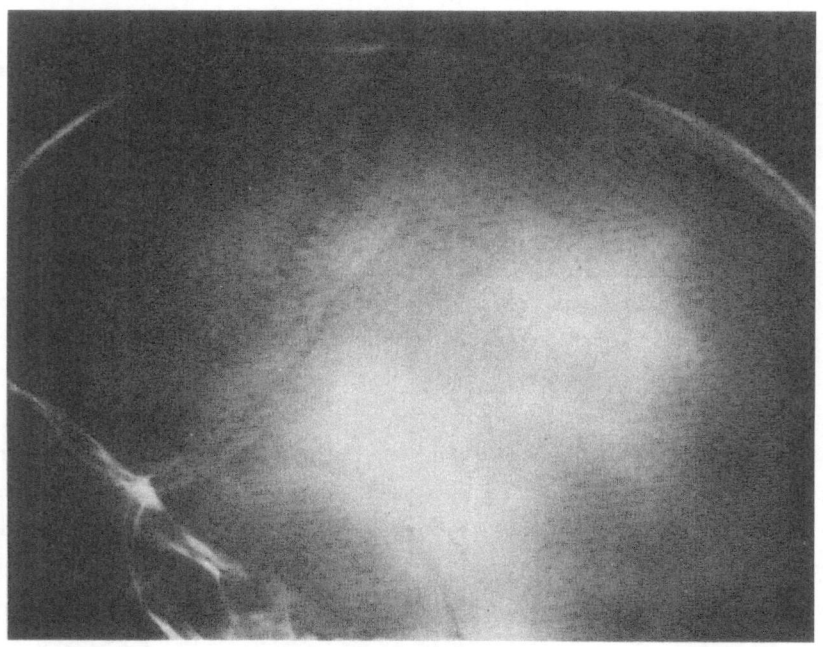

Figure 2: Neuroblastoma.   Plain skull.   There is diastasis of the
coronal suture.

CT was undertaken in 5 patients; all the tumours were of high
attenuation with the exception of the only intracerebral mass, which
had both high and low attenuation components (figure 3).   The tumours
enhanced markedly after intravenous contrast medium (figure 4); oedema
only surrounded the intracerebral tumour, but was not present in the
other cases.   All these tumours showed marked response to
radiotherapy (figure 5)

     There were 4 Ewing's sarcomas with multiple metastases to bones
and lungs.   A further case had a solitary intracerebral tumour, which
presented five years after the primary tumour had been apparently
cured.   There was excellent response to radiotherapy but a further
recurrence developed in the same region after another five years.   On
CT this was a high attenuation well-defined lesion in the right fronto-
parietal region with marked enhancement after intravenous contrast
medium and marked surrounding oedema (figure 6).

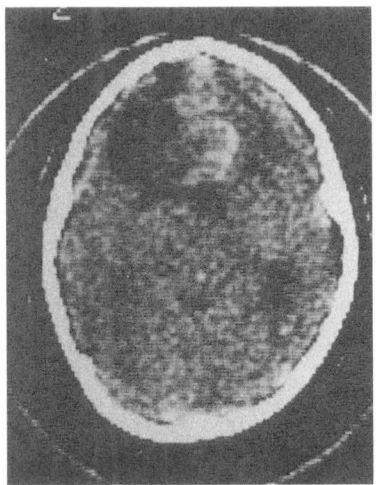

Figure 3. Neuroblastoma. Plain CT. There is a mixed high and low attenuation mass in left frontal pole extending across the midline

a 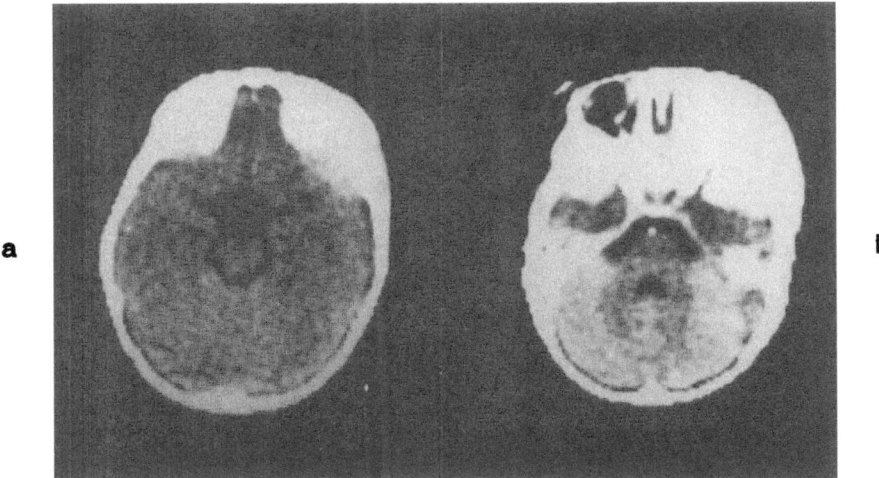 b

Figure 4. Neuroblastoma. Same case as figure 1. a) Plain scan. There is high attenuation mass peripherally placed near the tip of the right temporal lobe. b) slightly lower section after intravenous contrast medium. There is dense enhancement of the mass and a smaller enhanced mass is shown anterior to the left temporal lobe.

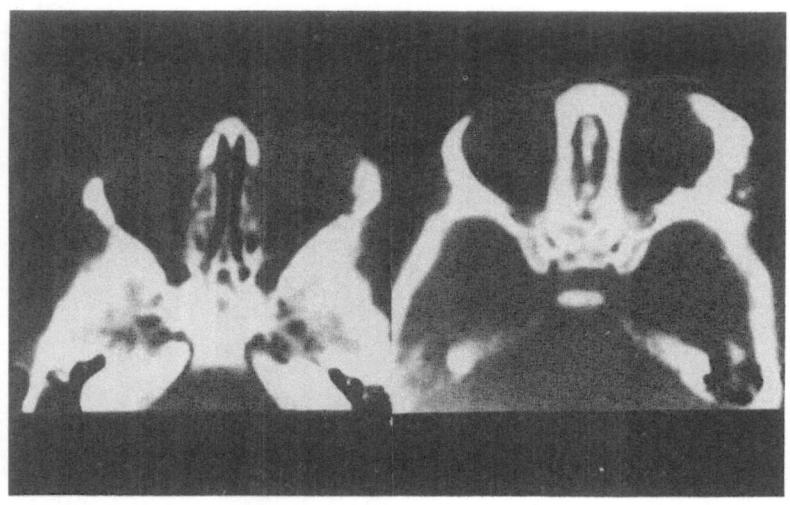

Figure 5. Neuroblastoma. Same case as figures 1 and 4. The tumour has regressed and the bone reconstituted following Deep X-ray Therapy

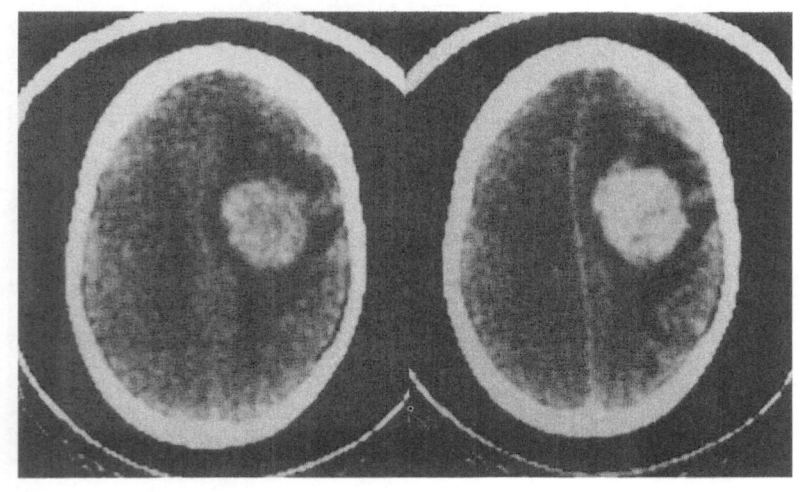

Figure 6. Ewing's sarcoma. a) Plain CT. There is a large high attenuation mass in the right fronto-parietal region with surrounding oedema. b) after contrast. There is dense homogeneous enhancement

In only one of the 40 Wilm's embryomas with metastases was there
an intracranial tumour. The patient was seen before the introduction
of CT Scanning, but plain films and angiograms showed a solitary cystic
tumour with increased vascularity primarily involving the temporal bone.

Of 12 metastatic rhabdomyosarcoma two were intracranial; in both
cases the lesions were solitary and no systemic metastases were found.
One involving the thalamus and mid brain was from a primary tumour in
the kidney; the other in the right lentiform nucleus (figure 7) was
from a parotid gland primary. Both were isodense with marked surrounding oedema and showed diffuse enhancement. There was apparently total
resolution of the lesions with radiotherapy (figure 8).

a 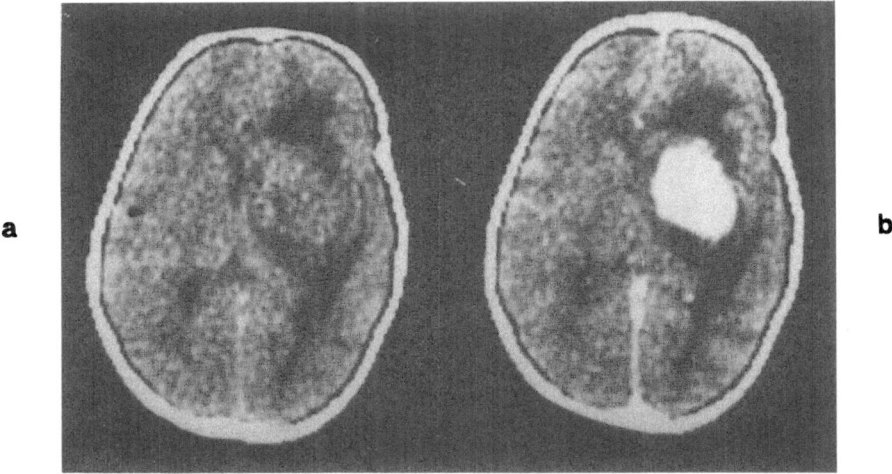 b

Figure 7. Rhabdomyosarcoma. a) Plain scan. There is a mass isodense
with brain in the right lentiform region with considerable surrounding
white matter oedema. b) after intravenous contrast. There is dense
homogeneous enhancement.

There were 11 hepatoblastomas with metastases. One presented in infancy
with multiple pulmonary masses and signs of a cerebral tumour before
CT Scanning was available. Angiography showed a solitary highly
vascular malignant frontal tumour.

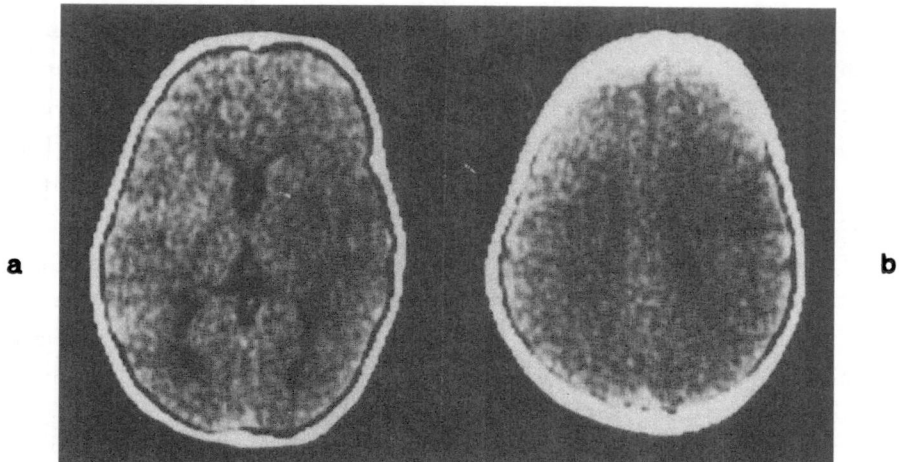

a   b

Figure 8: Same case, after irradiation. a and b) Plain scan. There
is only slight residual low attenuation without any mass effect.

The deposit in the case of the acute myeloid leukaemia was situated in
the right occipital lobe. It was of high attenuation with adjacent
oedema and showed marked enhancement (figure 9). Following radiotherapy

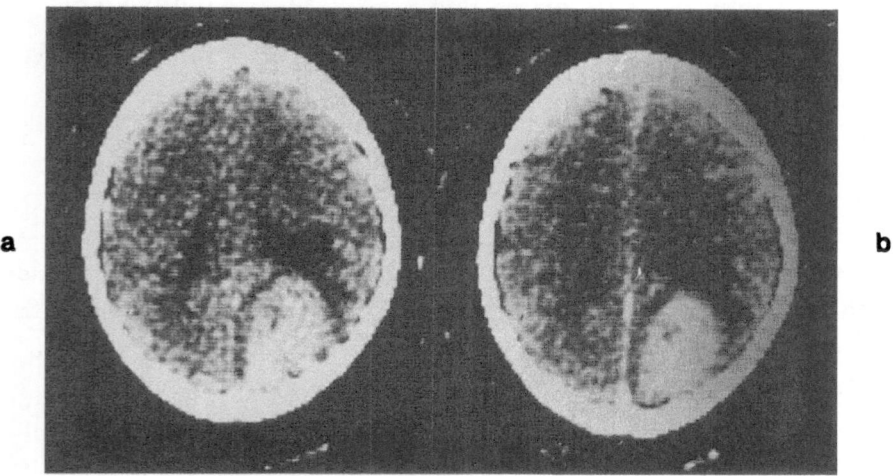

a   b

Figure 9: Leukaemia mass. a) Plain CT. There is a high attenuation
mass occupying the right occipital pole with oedema anterior to it,
b) after contrast. There is homogeneous enhancement.

the mass disappeared completely but recurred one year later. The
patient with acute lymphatic leukaemia had a low attenuation frontal
mass with surrounding enhancement; the diagnosis was confirmed by
biopsy. In both these cases there was C.S.F. findings of meningeal
leukaemia. In recent years the incidence of meningeal involvement has
been reduced to approximately 6% and these 2 patients therefore,
represent an incidence of less than 5% of cases with meningeal
leukaemia.

GROUP 2

Intracranial Metastases from the Nervous System

Twenty-one children with a previously proven primary cerebral neoplasm
developed intracranial metastases; their distribution is shown in
Table 2 . A medulloblastoma was the original tumour in 14 and in 7 of
the 11 patients scanned the metastases involved the subarachnoid space

a 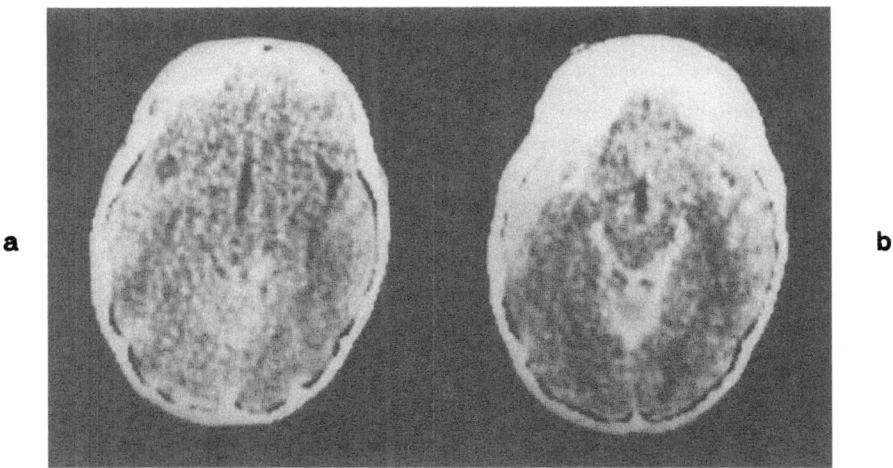 b

Figure 10. Medulloblastoma. a) Plain scan. There is effacement of the
basal cistern with abnormal high attenuation adjacent to the tentorial
hiatus. b) after contrast. There is abnormal enhancement in the same
regions.

either alone (figure 10) or as part of extensive involvement (figure 11);
only 3 had an intracerebral (figure 12) and one subependymal metastases
alone. In four cases the metastases were present at the time when the

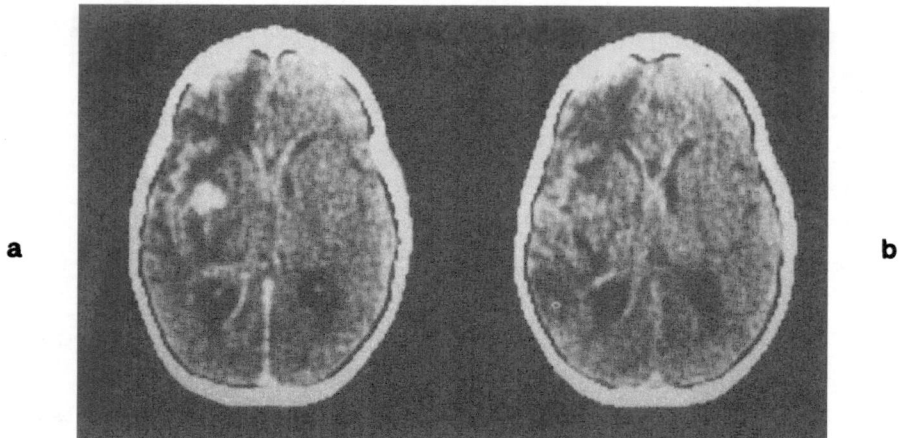

a   b

Figure 11: Medulloblastoma. a) Plain scan. b) after contrast. There
is high attenuation enhancing tumour around the margins of the left
lateral ventricle and right frontal horn in the left Sylvian fissure.
There is also a high attenuation enhancing nodule in the left lentiform
nucleus and there is surrounding oedema mainly in the white matter of
the left hemisphere.

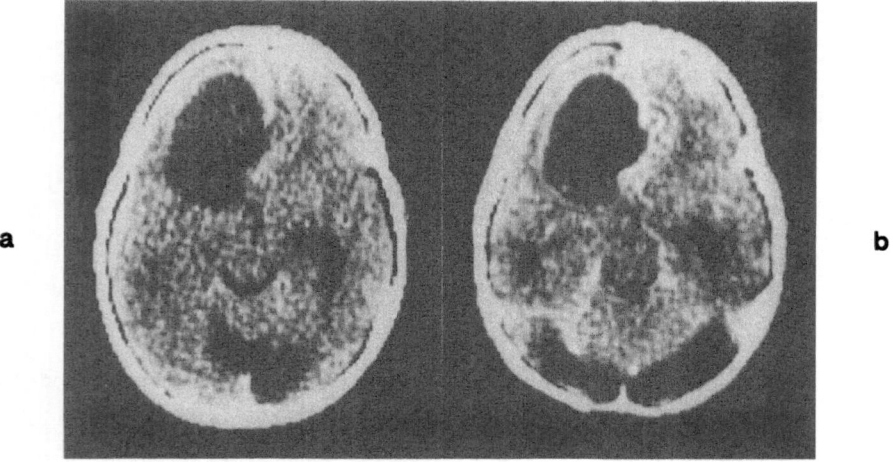

a   b

Figure 12: Medulloblastoma.   ᾳ) Plain scans. There is a large
left frontal mass of mixed attenuation with peripheral calcification and
central cystic or necrotic change.   b) Similar sections after
intravenous contrast. There is enhancement of the periphery of the cyst
and of the inferior solid component.

primary tumour was diagnosed, but in the others metastases presented up
to three years after the primary tumour. The intracerebral metastases
were of high attenuation on the plain scan. They were surrounded by
oedema of the white matter and following intravenous contrast medium
there was marked enhancement of the tumour tissue. Subependymal spread
distorted the contours of the ventricular system and was either isodense
with brain or of high attenuation on the plain scan, and enhanced
markedly (figure 13). Subarachnoid spread was sometimes difficult to
recognise on the plain scans. Most frequently there was effacement of
the subarachnoid cisterns by tumour isodense with brain; occasionally
there was high attenuation which was usually only seen adjacent to the
tentorium. There was invariably pronounced and extensive enhancement of
the tumour tissue (figure 10). Response to radiotherapy was often
dramatic but recurrence of the tumour was frequently demonstrated by
computed tomography in the same part of the subarachnoid space.

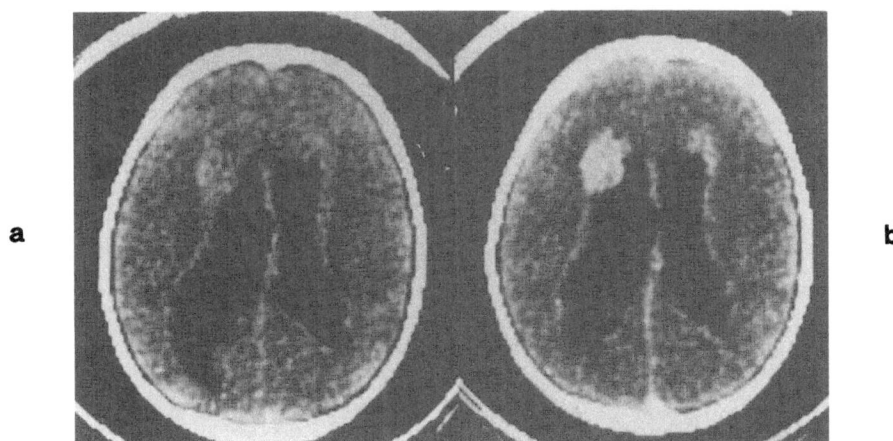

a   b

Figure 13. Medulloblastoma. a) Plain CT. There is high attenuation
periventricular tumour which has compressed the anterior horns and distorted the septum pellucidum. b) after contrast. There is marked
enhancement of the subependymal tumour tissue.

The pinealoma metastases projected into the dilated ventricles
(figure 14); one was isodense and the other was of slightly higher than
brain attenuation and both enhanced markedly. One ependymoma of the
IVth ventricle caused a large metastasis of mixed attenuation with

calcified and apparently cystic components (figure 15). The other had
a solitary isodense metastasis extending into the left lateral ventricle.
The solid components all enhanced.

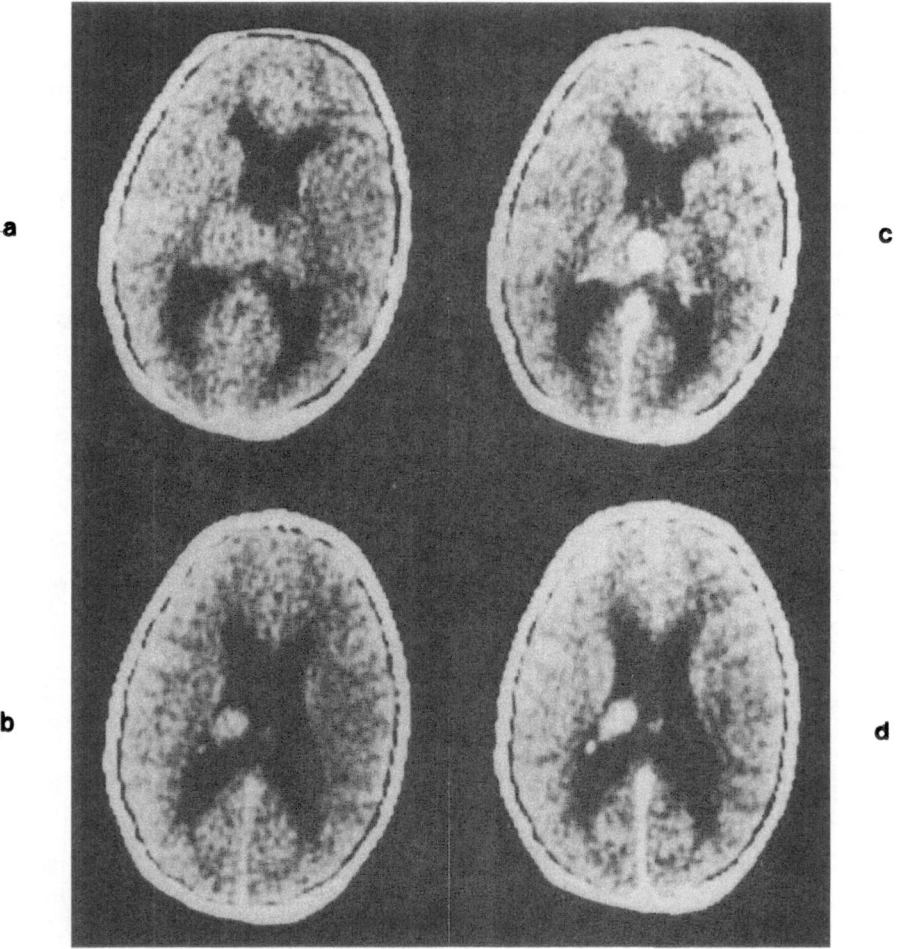

Figure 14. Pinealoma. a and b) Plain CT. c and d) after contrast.
There are enhancing masses of slightly higher than brain attenuation in
the pineal region and in the posterior part of the body of the left
lateral ventricle. There is symmetrical hydrocephalus.

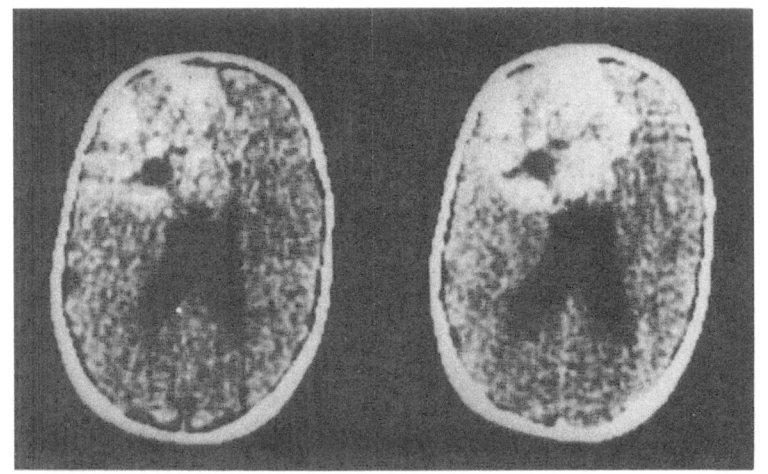

a

b

Figure 15. Ependymoma. a) Plain CT. b) after contrast. There is a large high attenuation, partly calcified enhancing tumour containing a small syst in the left frontal lobe extending across the midline. The anterior horns are effaced and the ventricles are dilated.

Both retinoblastomas caused metastases within the subarachnoid space. Masses adjacent to the posterior parts of the IIIrd ventricle in both cases were the probable cause of the hydrocephalus and in one there was a further isolated nodule in the suprasellar cistern (figure 16) a pattern simmulating that more commonly seen in pinealoma. Only one astrocytoma metastasised to the brain. It caused high attenuation periventricular masses mainly in the septum pellucidum which enhanced (figure 17).

GROUP 3

Spine from systemic

Only 4 patients presented with spinal cord involvement due to metastases from a systemic primary tumour. In each case the primary tumour was a neuroblastoma which was known to be separate and distant from the metastasis.

CT was not undertaken in any of thèse cases because it was considered at the time that the degree of mass effect on the spinal theca was best established by myelography. Three of the metastases were

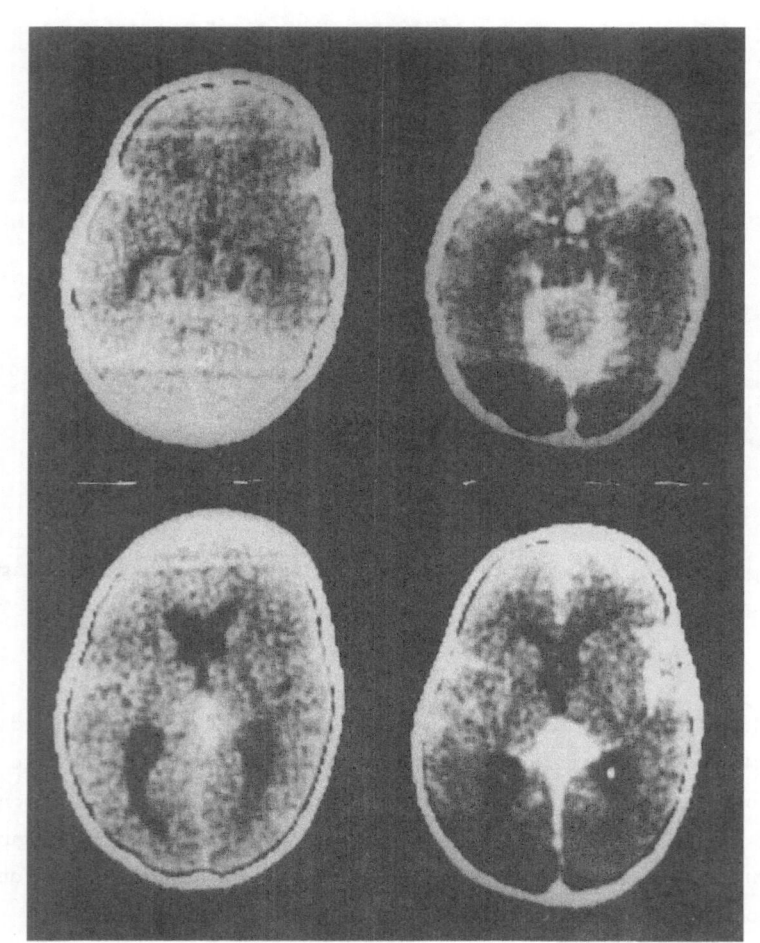

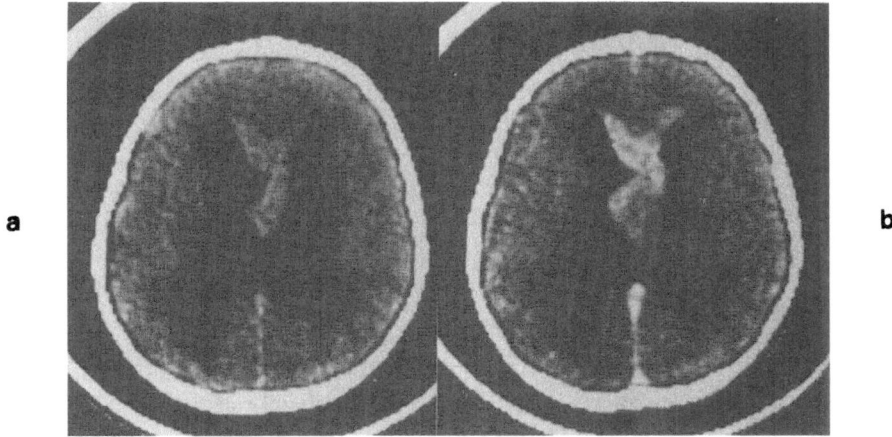

a   b

Figure 17. Astrocytoma. a) Plain CT. The septum pellucidum is widened and distorted by a high attenuation mass which encroaches upon the anterior horns and bodies. b) after contrast. There is extensive homogeneous enhancement

extradural; one was in the subarachnoid space and in all cases the presenting features were those of the metastasis.

GROUP 4

Systemic from nervous system

Three patients with a proven medulloblastoma subsequently developed extensive bony metastases (figure 18). In all of then hydrocephalus had previously been treated by a ventriculo-atrial shunt and in two of them cerebral metastases had been demonstrated. The time between the diagnosis of the primary tumour and the development of their bony metastases was one, two and five years respectively. The appearances of extensive osteoblastic skeletal metastases are among those which have been described in the literature (4 and 5).

GROUP 5

Spinal intrathecal from intracranial tumour (Table 3)

There were 11 cases. Nine were medulloblastomas; in seven of these the metastases were multiple, six involving the subarachnoid space and

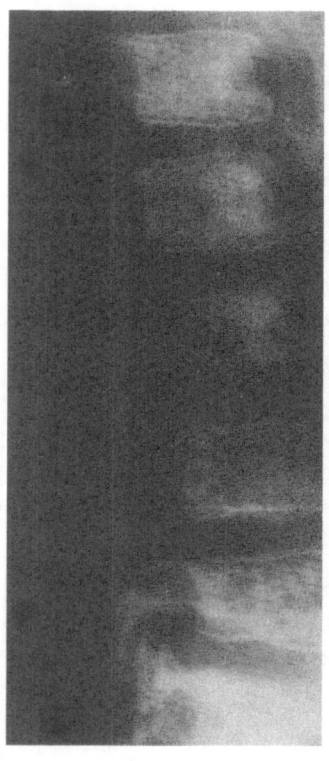

Figure 18: Medulloblastoma after ventriculo-atrial shunt, lateral projection of lumbar spine. There are multiple sclerotic lesions in the vertebral bodies.

one intramedullary with subarachnoid seedling. The other had an intramedullary mass alone. One patient was in a terminal state and was not submitted to myelography. The other two cases were pinealomas; both had multiple intramedullary metastases.

DISCUSSION

In our experience of 198 proven intracranial tumours diagnosed in the past 3 years, 28 (14%) demonstrated metastases on CT and in 2.5% the metastases were the presenting feature. These figures reflect the influence of computed tomography, as can be seen, from the fact that in the past 10 years only 44 intracranial metastases including the 28 referred to above have been recognised. Over the same period 17 children were diagnosed as having metastases involving the spinal cord. In 37 of these patients the intracranial metastases were of neural origin, 22 of them arising from the central nervous system and 15 from neuroblastomas. Only 7 metastases arose from other primary sites.

Eight of the patients with metastatic medulloblastomas have been scanned and in two of these the original diagnosis of the primary tumour was also made on computed tomography. During this 3 year period a total of 24 primary cases of medulloblastoma have been examined demonstrating the high incidence of intracranial metastatic disease in this condition. A very similar incidence is encountered in the ependymomas; though they are less frequent, two metastases and nine

primary tumours were scanned. Intracranial metastases from other
primary central nervous system tumours are less common, but are encountered from pinealomas, retinoblastomas and gliomas.

Intracerebral metastases from tumours outside the central nervous
system are less common however. Although there were a total of 22
intracranial metastases from systemic tumours, only 7 of these were
intracerebral including one neuroblastoma , one Ewing's sarcoma, one
hepatoblastoma, two rhabdomyosarcomas, one acute myeloid and one acute
lymphatic leukaemia. The Wilm's tumour and 14 of the 15 neuroblastomas
metastasised to the bone and dura and rarely appeared to invade the
brain substance.

During the ten years to 1979 analysis of the files of the Hospital
for Sick Children revealed the origin of the primary neoplasm in
patients with metastatic tumours in 236 cases (Table 4). Over 50% of
the metastases were of two histological types, neuroblastomas and
Wilm's sarcoma. The distribution of childhood metastases in the various
tumours presenting at Great Ormond Street is demonstrated in Table 5.
Intracerebral metastases from most primary tumours are relatively rare
and since the numbers of many histological types are small the incidence of 25% in Ewing's sarcoma and 20% in rhabdomyosarcoma in this
series quite probably is not a true reflection of the incidence of
such tumours.

The time interval between the diagnosis of the primary tumour and
the metastases varied widely. All the neuroblastomas, five of the 14
medulloblastomas and two of the 3 pinealomas had metastasized to the
nervous system at the time of diagnosis of the primary tumour. Although
this study encompasses a ten year period, during the past three years,
since CT has been available intracranial metastases have been the
presenting feature in 8 cases, 4 neuroblastomas, 2 medulloblastomas
and 2 pinealomas. In this time 198 proven intracranial tumours have
been scanned of which 28 (14%) were metastatic.

The incidence of metastases in other organs at the time of
diagnosis of the intracerebral metastases has also been assessed.
Apart from the 7 patients with bony metastases from medulloblastoma no
patient with primary central nervous system tumour had metastasised outside the central nervous system. The cranial lesion was the sole
metastasis in seven of the neuroblastomas and in the patients with
Wilm's sarcoma, rhabdomyosarcoma and leukaemias. In the other eight
neuroblastomas extensive bony involvement was present and in addition

there was visceral, marrow and pleural involvement in one case each; out of the entire series pulmonary metastases were only encountered in the patient with hepatoblastoma.

Prior to the use of cranial CT the diagnosis could only be made by angiography or encephalography, which was often not considered justified in children who were in poor general condition. Particularly, in those suffering from metastatic neuroblastoma only limited examination was undertaken; there was erosion of the sutures in five patients and focal bone destruction of the vault or facial bones in twelve.

In contradistinction to cranial CT body scanning has not facilitated the earlier detection of spinal metastases. Myelography was undertaken in all but two of the cases with symptoms of spinal involvement; the exceptions were a terminal case of medulloblastoma with a flaccid paralysis and a child with a neuroblastoma who had metastases on the cord at autopsy. All the other neuroblastoma metastases were extradural and two of the medulloblastomas and both pinealomas were intramedullary. At the time of the study myelography was considered to be the investigation of choice for assessing both the site and extent of intraspinal lesions.

Plain CT demonstrates paravertebral soft tissue masses and bone destruction and because of the axial plane of scanning it is of particular value in assessing parts of the vertebra; e.g. the lamina which are difficult to show with conventional radiographs. It also reveals the total extent of the tumour mass outside the theca but without metrizamide it is difficult to visualise details of thecal displacement.

Evaluation of the intrathecal structures is best achieved in most cases by conventional myelography with metrizamide. CT myelography performed soon after the conventional study, may give further localising information in the transverse plane about lesions which have been localised and may be particularly helpful in showing the upper limit of an almost conplete obstruction.

It has been suggested that CT myelography virtually eliminates the need for tomography and conventional myelography (6). We believe that this approach is impractical at present, except for the unusual case in which a lesion has already been well localised and a primary neoplasm confirmed; otherwise a large number of sections may be necessary because of the possibility of multiple lesions. As previously indicated we believe CT myelography is best used to supplement conventional studies rather than replace them.

Diagnosis by examination of the cerebro-spinal fluid alone was rarely used but the fluid was positive for tumour cells in 3 of the 6 cases of medulloblastoma in which detailed cytological studies were performed.

The cranial metastases in these children had fairly characteristic appearances. In all but three cases the tumours,whether intracerebral, subependymal, subarachnoid or extradural were either isodense or of high attenuation. The masses were usually well visualised even on the plain scan, especially the intracerebral tumours, which were surrounded by white matter oedema. Hydrocephalus was only present where the tumour masses were large enough to cause coning or in a position which compromised the C.S.F. pathways. Following intravenous contrast medium there was diffuse homogeneous enhancement of the whole tumour with two exceptions, the cystic metastasis from acute lymphatic leukaemia and the intracerebral metastasis of neuroblastoma, which was of mixed attenuation with patchy enhancement after contrast.

It has become increasingly evident that some tumours of childhood are associated with a higher than normal incidence of other malignant disease and in some there may be a family history. Two patients in this series, both with neuroblastomas, had one parent who had previously been treated for a retinoblastoma and a further child with a neuro-blastoma had a family history of two maternal cousins with lymphoma.

Some of the children in this series returned home overseas after treatment and in a number of cases the outcome of their disease is therefore not available. The overall follow-up is incomplete, but where information is available death within a few months was usual. Twelve of the patients with neuroblastoma are known to have died, six within five months of diagnosis and the longest interval between diag-nosis and death was 23 months. Five of the remaining six had extensive metastatic disease and therefore are presumed to have died. Metastatic medulloblastoma carries a similar prognosis, four of the patients dying within one month of presentation with their metastases, and a similar short survival occurred in the other tumours. Since the time interval between diagnosis and death irrespective of the treatment undertaken, is equally short and all patients were symtomatic when diagnosed it appears that the development of symptoms usually signifies a terminal state of the disease process.

The CT appearance of primary tumours has been extensively documented in children and the morphology is quite varied. The CT appearances in intracranial metastatic disease on the other hand, appears more consistent irrespective of the origin of the primary tumour or distribution of the metastases. High attenuation lesions with marked enhancement raise the possibility of metastatic disease. Furthermore, since some of the tumours have a predilection for particular sites it may be possible in these cases to suggest the origin of the metastasis.

In our practice malignant tumours of the central nervous system are treated either by total central nervous system irradiation extending beyond the limits of the tumour. Any further therapy would only be given for relief of symptoms due to recurrent or metastatic tumour. We do not perform routine follow-up scans on all cases since there is no evidence that treatment of asymptomatic tumours improves prognosis. However, CT is of great value in demonstrating the cause of any deterioration since this may be due to benign complications such as adhesive hydrocephalus and subdural effusions.

REFERENCES

1. Lee, FA, Paediatric X-ray diagnosis. Ed. Caffey 6th Edition. Lloyd Luke. p. 188, 1973

2. Globus, JH and T Meltzer, Metastatic tumours of the brain. Arch. Neurol. and Psych 48: 163-226, 1942

3. Störtebecker, TP, Metastatic tumours of the brain from a neuro-surgical point of view. J. Neurosurg. 11: 84-111, 1954

4. Debnam, JM and TW Staple, Osseous metastases from cerebellar medulloblastoma. Radiology 107: 363-366, 1973

5. Brutschin, P and GJ Culver, Extracranial metastases from medulloblastomas. Radiology 107: 359-362, 1973

6. Resjö, IM, DC Harwood Nash, CR Fitz and S Chuang, CT metrizamide myelography for intraspinal and paraspinal neoplasms in infants and children. Amer J Roentgen 132: 367-372, 1979

TABLE 1

Cranial and cerebral metastases from a systemic primary tumour

	Number	Time between 1° and 2°
Neuroblastoma	15	0 months (all)
Ewing's Sarcoma	1	5 years and 10 years
Wilm's Sarcoma	1	0 months
Rhabdomyosarcoma	2	2 months 3 years
Hepatoblastoma	1	0 months
Acute Myeloid Leukaemia	1	2 years
Acute Lymphatic Leukaemia	1	3 years

TABLE 2

Intracranial metastases from nervous system primary tumours

	Number	Time between 1° and 2°
Medulloblastoma	14	0 months (4) 0-1 year (6) 1 year (4)
Ependymoma	2	5 years 1 year
Retinoblastoma	2	3 years 2 years
Pinealoma	2	0 months 2 years
Astrocytoma	1	0 months

TABLE 3

Spinal intrathecal metastases from an intracranial primary tumour

	Number	Time between 1° and 2°
Medulloblastoma	9	0-1 year (7)
		2 years (2)
Pinealoma	2	0 months
		2 years

TABLE 4

Distribution of primary tumours in

236 childhood metastases

Neuroblastoma	89
Wilm's Sarcoma	40
Medulloblastoma	24
Teratoma	13
Hepatoblastoma	11
Rhabdomyosarcoma	10
Ewing's Sarcoma	4
Pinealoma	3
Astrocytoma	3
Ependymoma	2
Retinoblastoma	2
Miscellaneous Sarcoma	30
Miscellaneous Carcinoma	5

TABLE 5

Distribution of metastases (%)

	Bones	Lungs	Liver	Pleura	Craniospinal
Neuroblastoma	54	19	27	12	21
Wilm's Sarcoma	0	92	8	33	2.5
Medulloblastoma	12	0	0	0	100
Hepatoblastoma	0	9	0	0	9
Rhabdomyosarcoma	25	75	0	0	20
Ewing's Sarcoma	50	50	0	0	25

3. INDICATIONS FOR STEREOTACTIC BIOPSY IN BRAIN TUMOURS

D.A. Bosch

Introduction

Histological diagnosis is imperative for adequate
management of any mass lesion. For this reason stereotactic biopsy is indicated in all lesions of the brain in
which open surgery is not superior or is even impossible
for a variety of reasons.

Techniques

Brain surgery by biopsy is described only in some mono-
graphs (7,9) and various specialized papers.(3,4,8,12)
Stereotactic biopsy is performed with help of a
stereotactic device that is fixed on the patient's head.
X-rays in lateral and AP projections show the intracranial
space in a fixed relationship to the apparatus and after
visualization of the target (i.e. the mass lesion) on
these films its coördinates (x,y and z) can be calculated
according to the principles of the system. Visualization
can be done by angiography or ventriculography during the
stereotactic procedure, or, as is more often the case, by
superimposing already available films on the stereotactic
films with the appropriate corrections for differences in
magnification. Angiography is necessary for studying
the vascularity of the tumour and the anatomy
of the major vessels before doing any stereotactic
procedure.
In the Department of Neurosurgery in Groningen we perform

stereotactic biopsies using the Backlund spiral needle.(1)
This instrument is screwed into the target tissue after
stereotactically guided puncture through a burr-hole and
the overlying structures. The spiral has a length of 12 mm
and a diameter of 1.2 mm. As a standard procedure we take
3 samples along the puncture track if the tumour location
permits this: one before reaching, one in and one behind
the calculated target. (See fig. 1: points 1,2 and 3) If
still more tissue is requested by the pathologist, who
studies the samples during the procedure, another 3
samples are taken from a parallel track that is realized
by slightly altering the z - coördinate. (fig. 1:
points 4,5 and 6) In fig. 2 a biopsy needle is shown on
X-ray.The tissue samples with this type of biopsy are
normally of excellent quality for histological examination
(fig. 3 and 4) and for this reason we prefer the spiral
needle to the conventional aspiration needles.

Indications

In the management of patients in good general condition,-
i.e., able to survive long enough to justify radiation
and/or chemotherapy in the case of a treatable tumour or
metastasis - stereotactic biopsy should be performed
whenever open surgery with at least bulk resection are
not feasible. Broadly there are in the treatment of mass
lesions areas of the brain which are accessible to open
surgery (fig. 5) and other areas which are not.(fig. 6)
In between are many situations in which an individual
decision has to be taken; mainly depending on the
anatomical borders of the process and the clinical state
of the patient. Since computerized axial tomography
became available, the decision to perform a stereotactic
biopsy has been made more frequently than previously.
In this context, the following advantages of CT-scanning
compared to angiography and isotope scanning deserve
special attention.

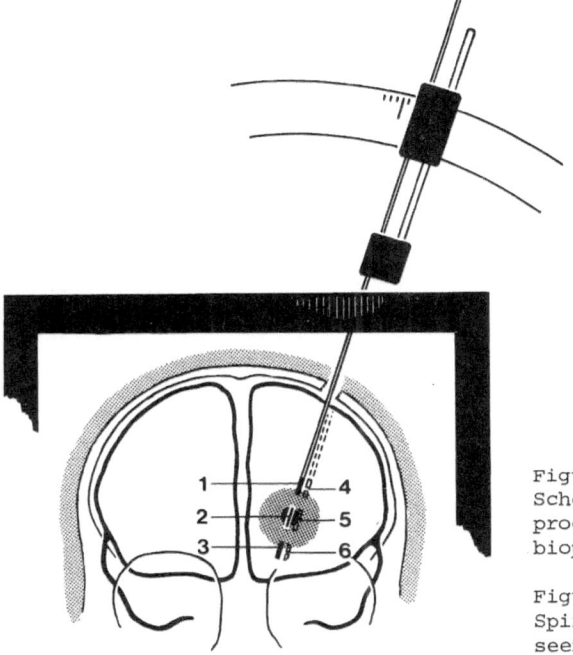

Figure 1.
Schematic drawing of sampling
procedure in stereotactic
biopsy

Figure 2.
Spiral needle in target as
seen on X-ray

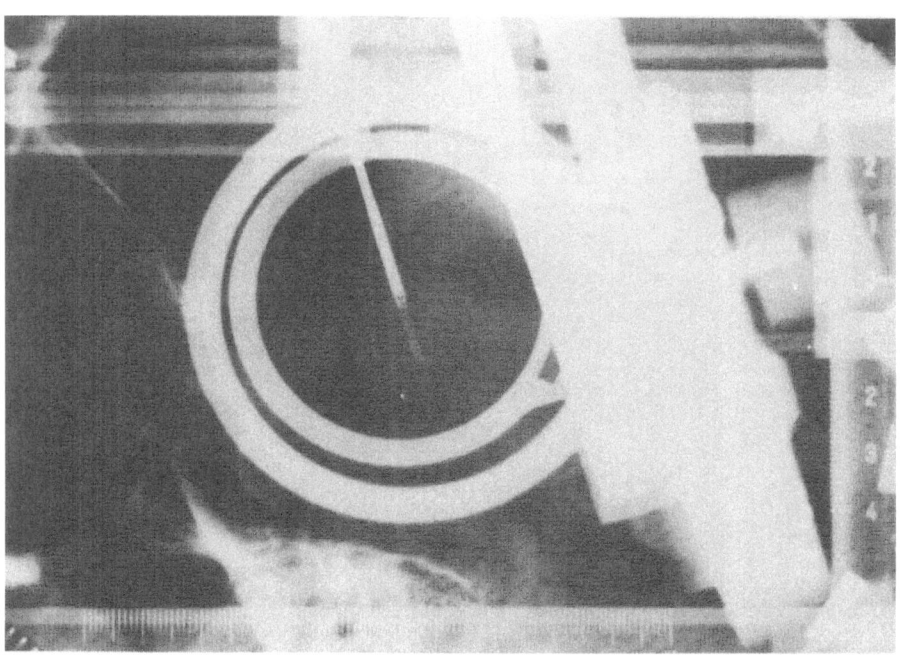

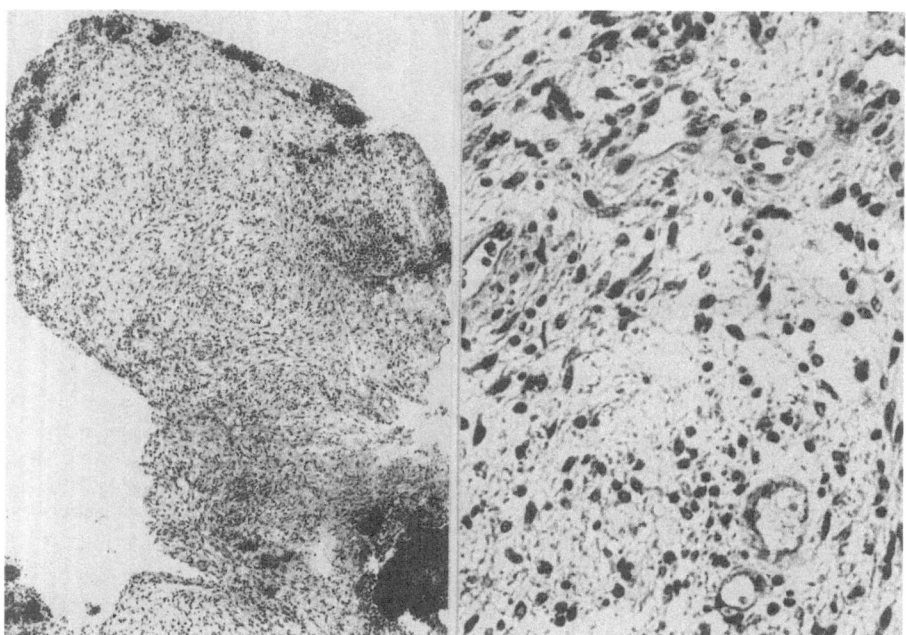

Figure 3. Astrocytoma, H & E, magnifications: 44,8x and 280x

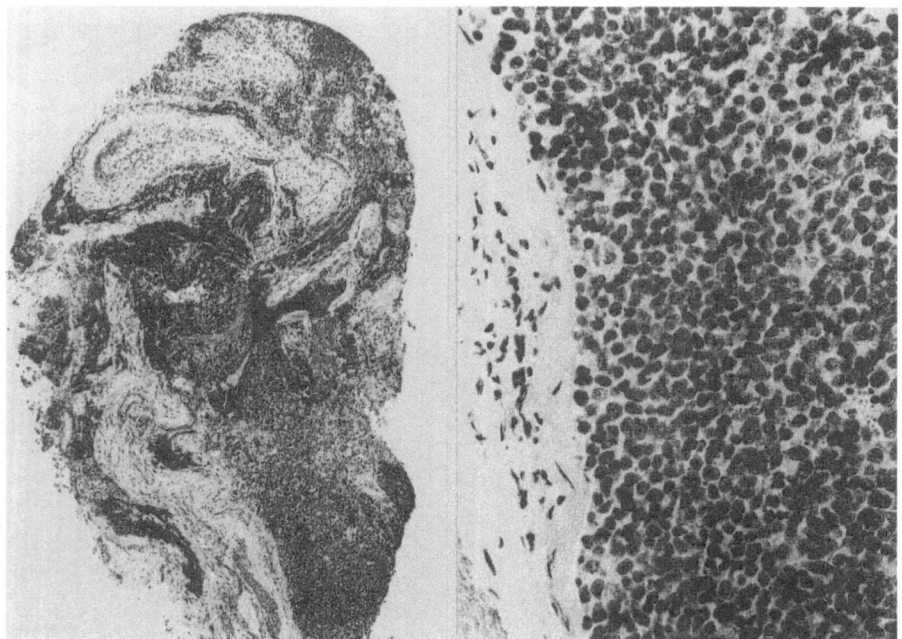

Figure 4. Carcinoma metastasis, H & E, magnifications: 44,8x and 280x

-1- clearer delineation of the medial border of the process
    which allows pre-operative assessment of amenability
    to open surgery. (example: butterfly tumour)
-2- detection of as yet small lesions in the midline
    which could be treated by radiotherapy if histological
    proof of radiosensitivity has been obtained (example:
    dysgerminoma (8)
-3- detection of the cystic nature of midline tumours
    allows treatment by simple puncture and evacuation
    (example: colloid cyst of the third ventricle (2)
-4- higher resolution of the imaging process leads to
    earlier and better visualization of multiple mass
    lesions (example: metastases)
-5- detection of intracerebral manifestations of systemic
    or generalized malignant disease that might be
    treated preferably by non-surgical means (examples:
    leukemia (13), lymphoma (6).

From the situations mentioned above it is clear that the
information provided by CT-scanning leads to more
indications for stereotactic biopsy as an imperative step
in the management of patients harbouring intracerebral
mass lesions. In general, the strongest presumption of
the lesions's nature - as given by the latest generation
of CT-scanners - is no substitute for histological
evidence. In discussing the indications for stereotactic
biopsy in brain tumours one can distinguish four different
groups of patients. (see tables 1 and 2)

A. Patients without a previous history of tumour and who
   present with a single intracerebral mass lesion. In
   general, this is the case in primary tumours of the
   brain, but sometimes a secondary (still solitary)
   tumour will be encoutered in a patient with an unknown
   primary malignancy elsewhere. Open craniotomy should be
   carried out whenever the possibility exists of removing
   a lesion, as even bulk resection of a glioma is
   preferable to biopsy if radiotherapy is to be given
   afterwards. Only in cases in which complete or bulk

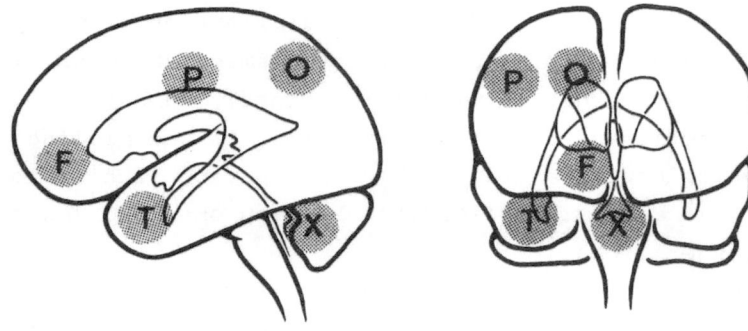

peripheral large tumours ▶ BULK RESECTION

Figure 5.

Table 1.   Indications for stereotactic biopsy in brain
            tumours in cases without known primary tumour
            elsewhere

mass lesion number	surgical technique	histology
1	removable: craniotomy	glioma lymphoma
	not removable: biopsy, if further treatment is justified	metastasis miscellaneous
≥ 2	biopsies, if further treatment is justified	metastases multiple primaries miscellaneous

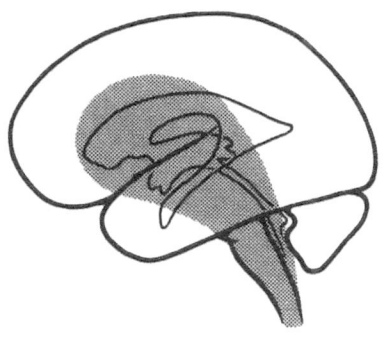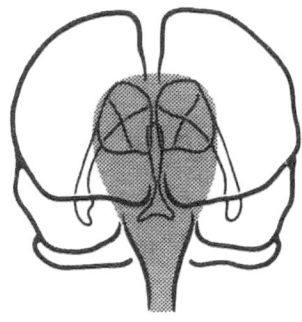

all sizes midline tumours ▶ STEREOTACTIC BIOPSY

Figure 6.

Table 2. Indications for stereotactic biopsy in brain
tumours in cases with known primary tumour
elsewhere, but without other metastatic spread.

mass lesion number	surgical technique	histology
1	removable: craniotomy	metastasis
		second tumour
	not removable: biopsy, if further treatment is justified	non-neoplastic disease
		miscellaneous
≧ 2	biopsies, if further treatment is justified	metastases
		non-neoplastic disease
		miscellaneous

resection is impossible is stereotactic biopsy the
procedure of choice. Therefore, a stereotactic biopsy
is performed only in midline tumours and in very large
but diffusely growing hemispherical processes (for
example: gliomatosis cerebri).

B. Patients without a previous history of tumour and who
present with multiple intracerebral mass lesions.
These patients are of course suspected to bear a
malignancy elsewhere in the body and should be
investigated thoroughly for this. However, screening
is time consuming and it is not uncommon for no
primary tumour to be found. Also, previous immunosuppressive treatment (as in transplant procedures (11)
may lead to 'de novo' development of brain lymphomas.
As in these cases the tumours only occasionally permit
open surgery because of their multiplicity, we perform
a stereotactic biopsy of one or two of the lesions in
order to assist the oncologist by providing him with
the histological characteristics of the process.

C. Patients with a known primary tumour elsewhere and who
present with a single intracerebral mass lesion, but
without signs of metastasis elsewhere in the body.
Their management is dependent on site and on size of
the lesion. If at all possible an open craniotomy
should be performed to resect the lesion in toto. If
not, stereotactic biopsy is required to ascertain the
pathology of the tumour, since the lesion is not
always a metastasis of the primary tumour. With the
improvement in tumour therapy (radiation and
chemotherapy) survival tends to increase so that, at
the same time, the incidence of a second tumour
increases.(5,10) Also, the frequency of non-neoplastic
mass lesions in the brain is higher in patients
treated for malignancies. Mycotic and other abscesses
can be diagnosed stereotactically and treated
afterwards by drainage and the appropriate antibiotics.

D. Patients known to have a primary tumour elsewhere and

who present with multiple mass lesions in the brain
without other metastatic spread. A decision should be
made as to the desirability of any further treatment
on the basis of the patient's condition and the
characteristics of the primary tumour. The
differentiation between a metastatic and non-neoplastic
process is made most easily by stereotactic biopsy.
In general, however, further treatment is almost always
based on the histological characteristics of the
primary tumour: radiation and/or chemotherapy are
started if the tumour is suspected to be sensitive.
If not, open surgery might be attempted in the rare
case that presents with two resectable lesions.

Acknowledgements. the author is greatly indebted to
Professor E.J.Ebels for histological investigations
and to Mr. Douwe Buiter for excellent technical
assistance.

References

1. Backlund, EO, A new instrument for stereotaxic brain tumour biopsy. Acta Chir Scand 137:825-827, 1971

2. Bosch, DA, T Rähn, and EO Backlund, Treatment of Colloid Cysts of the third ventricle by stereotactic aspiration. Surg Neurol 9:15-18, 1978

3. Conway, LW, Stereotactic Biopsy of deep Intracranial Tumors. In: Current Techniques in operative neurosurgery, Schmidek, HH, and H Sweet (eds.), New York, Grune & Stratton, 187-198, 1977

4. Edner, G, Stereotaxic brain tumor biopsy-five year's experience. Proceedings of the 26th annual meeting. Acta Neurochir 31:261, 1975

5. Getaz, EP, Second malignant neoplasms in Hodgkin's Disease. Cancer Chemother Pharmacol 2:143-145, 1979

6. Henry, JM, RR Heffner, SH Dillard, KM Earle, and RL Davis, Primary malignant lymphomas of the central nervous system. Cancer 34: 1293-1302, 1974

7. Leksell, L, Stereotaxis and Radiosurgery. An operative System. Springfield Ill, Thomas, 1971

8. Pecker, J, JM Scarabin, JM Brücher, and B Vallée, Apport des techniques stéréotaxiques au diagnostic et au traitement des tumeurs de la région pinéale. Rev Neurol (Paris) 134: 287-294, 1978

9. Pecker, J, JM Scarabin, JM Brücher, and B Vallée, Démarche stéréotaxique en neurochirurgie tumorale. Paris: Les Éditions Médicinales Pierre Fabre, 1979

10. Schoenberg, BS, BW Christine, and JP Whisnant, Nervous system neoplasms and primary malignancies of other sites. Neurology 25: 705-712, 1975

11. Schneck, SA, and I Penn, De-novo brain tumors in renal transplant recipients. Lancet i: 983-986, 1971

12. Waltregny, A, V Petrov, and J Brotchi, Serial stereotaxic biopsies. Acta Neurochir Suppl 21: 221-226, 1974

13. Wolk, RW, SR Masse, R Conklin, and EJ Freireich, The incidence of central nervous system leukemia in adults with acute leukemia. Cancer 33: 863-869, 1974

4. IMMUNE DEPOSITS IN SURAL NERVE BIOPSIES FROM PATIENTS WITH PARANEOPLASTIC POLYNEUROPATHY

T.M. Feltkamp-Vroom, B.W. Ongerboer de Visser, C.A. Feltkamp

INTRODUCTION

Polyneuropathy, as a remote effect of malignant disease, is poorly understood. Metabolic factors, deficiency states and viral infection have been considered in the pathogenesis(1). Vasculitis (2), paraproteinaemia in myeloma (3) and immunopathologic factors are also reported as a cause for paraneoplastic neurological syndromes. The following data prompted us to study sural nerve biopsies with light, immunofluorescence and electron microscopy. Firstly, were proven circulating immune complexes found in patients with rheumatoid arthritis and Felty's syndrome with polyneuropathy in whom studies of sural nerve biopsies revealed immune deposits in the perineural membrane which consisted of immunoglobulin M (IgM) and thirdcomplement component (C3) (own observation). Secondly, recently, circulating immune complexes have been demonstrated in carcinoma of uterine cervix (4), gastrointestinal tract (5), and the immune-complex induced glomerulopathies of neoplasia (6). From these data it seemed attractive to postulate that immune complexes might play a role in the induction of polyneuropathy in patients with malignant diseases.

In the present study sural nerve biopsies were taken from 5 patients with malignant disease showing paraneoplastic polyneuropathy.

STUDY GROUP.

Five patients with various types of malignant disease and severe progressive polyneuropathy were selected for the study.

Neurological examination showed symptoms and signs of polyneuropathy (table 1) confirmed by electromyography.

Table 1

Clinical data of patients with paraneoplastic polyneuropathy.

Case number	Sex	Age in years	Malignancy	Polyneuropathy
1	M	28	Hodgkin	Sensorimotor
2	F	53	Oatcell carcinoma	Sensorimotor
3	M	57	Bronchial carcinoma	Sensory
4	M	63	Mouth floor carcinoma	Sensorimotor
5	F	65	Breast carcinoma	Sensory

In table 2 the intervals are summarized between the discovery of the tumour and the polyneuropathy, and that between the onset of the neuropathy and the biopsy.

Table 2

Intervals between discovery of malignancy and onset of polyneuropathy and between the onset of the polyneuropathy and the biopsy.

Case number	Interval between malignancy and neuropathy	Interval between neuropathy and malignancy	Interval between neuropathy and biopsy
1	3 years		5 months
2		3 months	6 months
3	2 months		3 months
4	8 years		7 years
5		2 months	4 months

All 5 patients had normal immunoglobulin levels in the serum and normal renal function. No paraproteinaemia was found.

In 2 of the 5 patients, the polyneuropathy preceded the discovery of the malignancy and in the other 3 the malignant disease was already known when the polyneuropathy became evident.

Twenty sural nerve samples taken at autopsy from patients without complaints of polyneuropathy served as controls. They had various diseases among which were malignancies, Wernicke encephalopathy, alcoholic liver disease, pneumonia and cerebral haemorrhage.

METHODS

The sural nerve biopsies were cut in 4 parts: snap-frozen in liquid nitrogen for immunofluorescence; fixed in buffered 4% formaldehyde (pH 7.2) for light microscopy; fixed in buffered paraformaldehyde- glutaraldehyde mixture of Karnovsky (7) for electron microscopy and lastly fixed for 20 min. in 1% paraformaldehyde- 0.05% glutaraldehyde for immunoelectron microscopy (8). Subsequently this part of the tissue was rinsed for 80 min. in 0.1% bovine serum albumin in phosphate buffered saline (pH 7.2) and then snapfrozen in liquid nitrogen. The light microscopy was performed on 4μm paraplast embedded sections, which were stained with haematoxylin-eosin, Gomori's trichrome, Bodian and Congo Red. The immunofluorescence procedure was the same as described before (9). The antisera used were labeled anti human IgG, IgM and IgA and anti C3 purchased from Dakopatts (Denmark), while anti first complement component q (Clq) purchased from the Central Laboratory of the Netherlands Red Cross Blood Transfusion Service was used in the indirect technique. Of all tissue specimens thin sections were prepared for electron micro-scopy according to routine methods. Thick (8 μm) frozen sections, cut from the frozen blocks prepared for immunoelectron microscopy, were attached to glycerinated coverslips and incubated with rabbit anti human IgM and peroxydase-labeled horse anti rabbit immunoglobulin anti-serum as a second layer. After reaction with diamino-benzidine and H_2O_2 the sections were postfixed with osium tetroxide and embedded in Epon and Araldite.

Parts with a positive dark brown reaction product and corresponding parts of control-incubated sections were selected with light microscopy and thin-sectioned. Elution studies were done by eluting cryostat sections from the tissue of the 5 patients in an acid citrate buffer (pH 3.2) for 30 min. Subsequently the sections were rinsed with phosphate buffered saline (pH 7.2) and incubated with anti IgM, anti IgG and anti C3 respectively.

RESULTS.

Light microscopy revealed no abnormalities in cases 1 and 3. In the neural tissue of the other 3 patients, myelin vacuolation and varying degrees of loss of myelinated fibres were seen. Congo Red positive material was not observed in any of the tissues. All nerve biopsies showed immune deposits as observed by immunofluorescence microscopy. They varied from faint granular IgM (fig. 1a) in the inner part of the perineural membrane together with very little C3 (fig. 1b) to heavy confluent granular layers of IgM (fig. 2a) with some C3 (fig. 2b) and Clq in the perineural membrane. No vascular immune deposits were observed in the endo- and epineural tissue. Faint diffuse IgG and IgA were present in the endoneural tissue of the 5 patients here described, as well as in that of the control tissues. IgM, C3 and Clq were not however found in any of the controls. Elution studies of the sural nerve sections only resulted in a slightly weaker presence of IgM but no IgG became detectable in the perineural membrane. Electron microscopy of routinely embedded biopsies of all cases with polyneuropathy showed discrete deposits of electron dense material between and against the basement membranes of the perineural cells, especially of the innermost layers (fig. 3): The structure of these deposits varied from amorphous to fibrillar (12-15 nm diameter), sometimes with a definite periodicity of about 100 nm (fig.3). In a few places the fibrils were more criss-cross arranged, giving the deposits an amyloid like appearance. Locally the deposits formed a continuous layer.

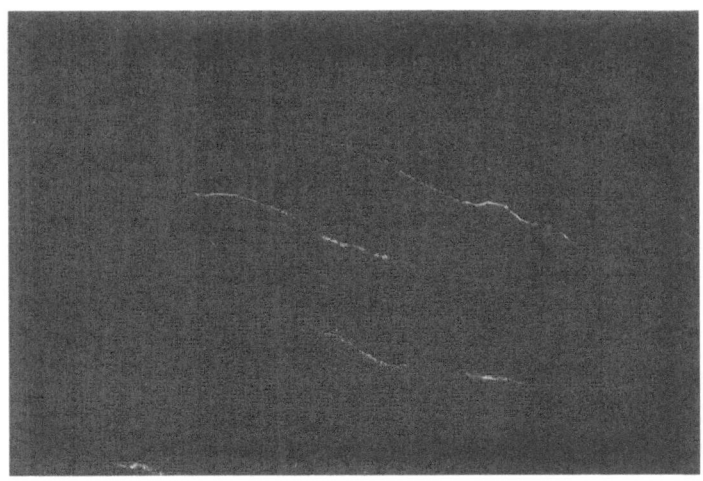

a

b

Fig. 1a: Sural nerve cryostat section incubated with rabbit
anti human IgM (x 80). Faint, granular to confluent deposition of IgM is seen in the perineural
membrane.

Fig. 1b: Sural nerve cryostat section of the same patient
as shown in fig. 1a incubated with rabbit anti
human C3 (x 200). Local, very faint deposition is
seen in the perineural membrane.

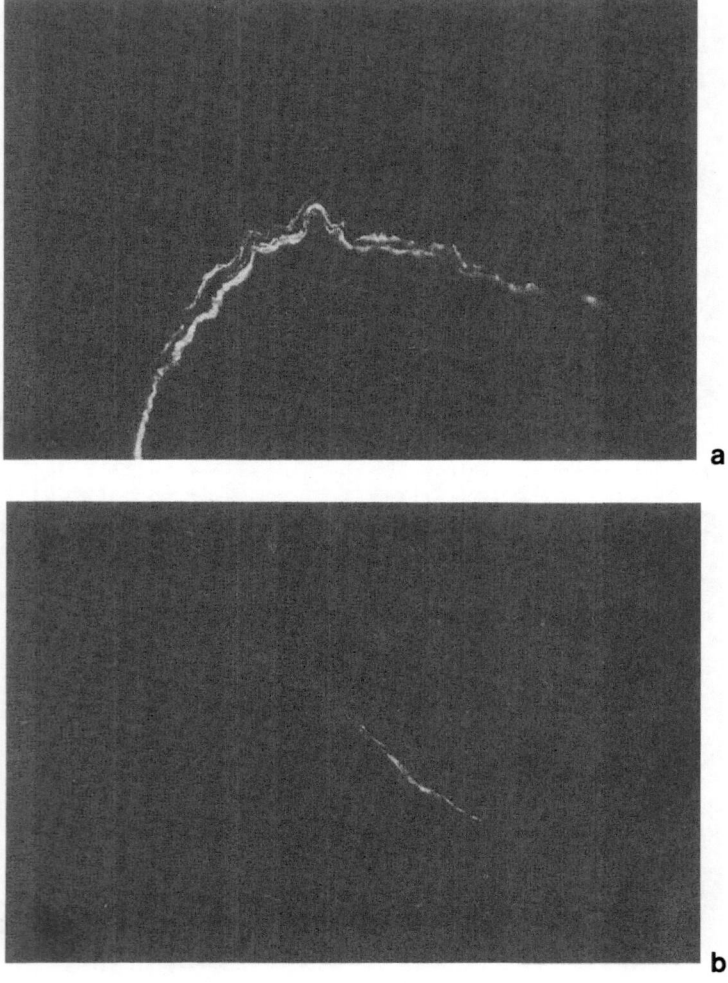

Fig. 2a: Sural nerve cryostat section incubated with
rabbit anti human IgM (x 320). Heavy, confluent
layer of IgM is present in the perineural
membrane.

Fig. 2b: Sural nerve cryostat section of the same patient
as shown in fig. 2a incubated with rabbit anti
human C3 (x 200). A faint, confluent deposition
of C3 is shown in the perineural membrane.

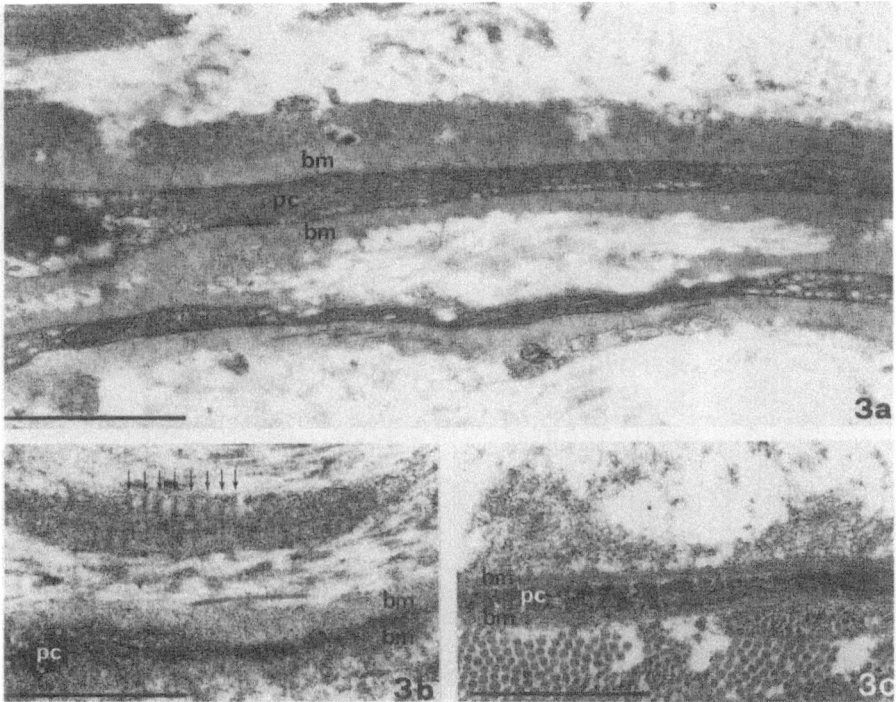

Fig. 3   Deposits of material against and between the base-
         ment membranes (bm) of perineural cells (pc). The
         deposits are amorphous (3a), granular (3b) or
         fibrillar (3c) and sometimes show a regular periodi-
         city (3b, arrows) x 24,000.

50

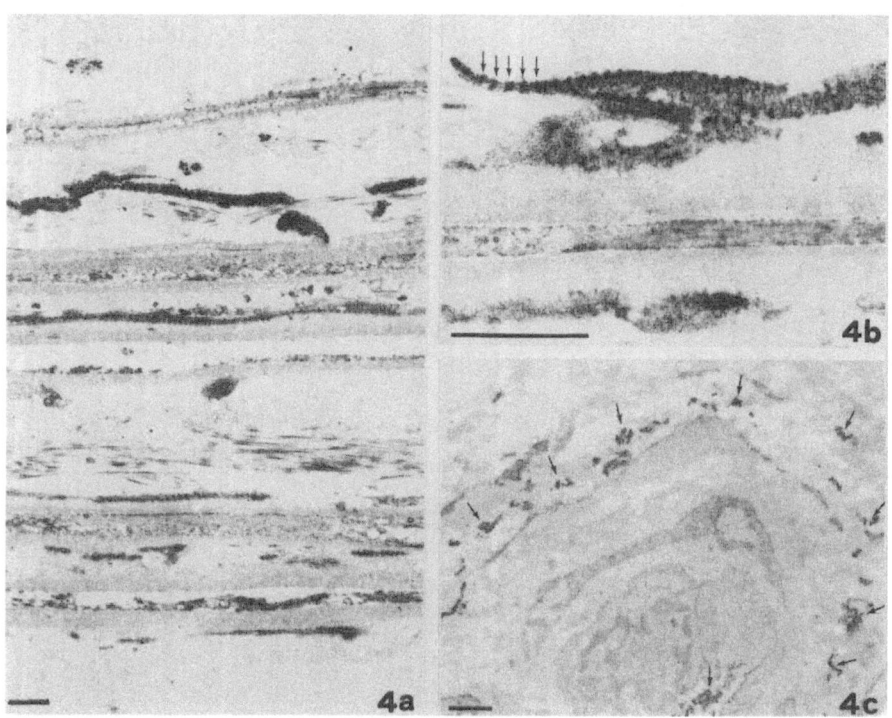

Fig. 4 The presence of IgM detected by an indirect immuno-
peroxydase technique. IgM positive deposits can
show a regular periodicity (4b, arrows); they are
also present in and around small endoneural vessels
(4c, arrows). a x 6,080; b x 18,200; c x 5,600.

With immunoelectron microscopy it became clear that the
deposits were positive for IgM (fig. 4). Moreover, small
IgM deposits were observed around some small endoneural
capillaries (fig. 4C).

The presence of C3 was not investigated by immunoelectron microscopy so that we were unable to see whether
these IgM deposits were combined with C3. By immunofluorescence microscopy, however, no C3-IgM deposits
were found in these vessel walls. A finding which suggests
that only very small deposits could have been present here.

DISCUSSION.

In the sural nerves of 5 patients with paraneoplastic
neuropathy, IgM in varying degrees of density, and C3 to a
lesser extent, could be identified in the perineural
membrane by the immunofluorescence technique. The presence
of IgM deposits was confirmed by immunoelectron microscopy.
Moreover, by this technique, small IgM deposits were seen
occasionally in the endoneural vascular walls.
This latter finding suggests that these small immune
deposits in the vessel walls might be induced by circulating immune complexes. Recently various authors described
circulating immune complexes in patients with malignant
diseases (4-6). One (5) of them reported that in a high
precentage of these patients the immune complexes consisted
of IgM and antigen.
Therefore it is possible that the IgM deposits in vessel
walls found in this study correspond with the presence of
immune complexes consisting of neoplastic antigen and IgM
as an antibody. That the presence of circulating immune
complexes can lead to small IgM· C3 deposits in vascular
walls is also described by Morris et al. (10) who found
such immune deposits in the skin of patients with systemic
lupus erythematosus.
Since elution of crystat sections did not lead to the
detection of IgG, which might act as antigen to IgM, it is
not likely that a mixed immunoglobulin complex in the serum,
consisting of IgG-IgM is the cause of the IgM-C3 perineural
deposits. Also, the normal immunoglobulin level of the

serum, and the absence of a paraproteinaemia, do not
suggest that   abnormal immunoglobulin(s), as causative
agent for a primairy amyloidosis, is present here. Besides
the electron microscopic features and the negative Congo
read staining are against amyloid deposits.

From many studies it is known that by the activation of
complement immune complexes induce an increase of vascular
permeability by which deposition and permeation of serum
proteins become possible in the vascular and perivascular
tissues. By this mechanism it is possible that IgM, which
is a high molecular protein,   once passed through the
vessel wall, spreads into the endoneural tissue and
becomes trapped in the perineural membrane which acts
as a filter barrier (11). When present in a high concentration it is possible that IgM can be found in peculiar
configurations as described for glomerular capillaries (12).
Further study is needed to elucidate the induction and
the significance of these immune deposits in nerve tissue
of patients with paraneoplastic polyneuropathy.
Acknowledgment.

We thank Mrs. J. Thomassen-Heins, Miss H. Spiele, Mrs. B.
Jorritsma-Bijham and Mr. G. Scholte for expert technical
assistance.

REFERENCES:

1. Bruyn, G.W., Carcinomatous polyneuropathy. In handbook of Clinical Neurology. Vol. 38, pp 679-693, 1979

2. Johnson, P.C., Rolak, L.A., Hamilton, R.H. and Laguna, J.F., Paraneoplastic vasculitis of nerve: A remote effect of cancer. Ann Neurol. 45: 437-444, 1979.

3. Dayan, A.D., Ulrich, H. and Gardner-Thorpe, C. Peripheral neuropathy and myeloma. J. Neurol. 14: 21-35, 1971.

4. Seth, P., Balachiandran, N., Melaninga, A.N. and Kumar, R. Circulating immune complexes in carcinoma of uterine cervix. Clin. exp. Immunol. 38: 77-82, 1979.

5. Kapsopoulou-Dominos, K. and Anderer, F.A. Circulating carcinoembryonic antigen immune complexes in sera of patients with carcinomata of the gastrointestinal tract. Clin. exp. Immunol. 35: 190-195, 1979.

6. Eagen, J.W. and Lewis, E.J. Editorial review on Glomerulopathies of neoplasia. Kidney Int. 11: 297-306, 1977.

7. Karnovsky M.J. A.formaldehyde-glutaraldehyde fixative of high osmolality for use in electron microscopy. J. Cell. Biol. 27: 137a-138a, 1965.

8. Meuwissen, S.J.M., Feltkamp-Vroom, Th.M., de la Rivière, A., v.d. Borne, A.E.G.Kr. and Tytgat, G.N. Analysis of the lymphoplasmacytic infiltrate in Crohn's disease with special reference to identification of lymphocyte-subpopulations. Gut 17: 770-780, 1976.

9. Smit, J.W., Meyer, C.J.L.M., Decary, F.and Feltkamp-
    Vroom, Th.M.
    Paraformaldehyde fixation in immunofluorescence and
    immuno-electron microscopy. J. immunol. Meth.6: 93-98,
    1974.

10. Morris, R.J., Guggenheim, S.J., McIntosh, R.M., Rubin,
    R.L. and Kohler, P.F.
    Simultaneous immunologic studies of skin and kidney in
    systemic lupus erythematosus. Arthritis Rheumatism 22:
    864-870, 1979.

11. Söderfeldt, B., Olsson, Y. and Kristensson, K.
    The perineurium as a diffusion barrier to protein
    tracers in human peripheral nerve. Acta Neuropath.
    (Berl.) 25: 120-126, 1976.

12. Thiele, J., Kühn, K., Zobl, H. and Krull, P.
    Die frühen morphologischen Veränderungen der mensch-
    lichen Niere bei Paraproteinämie. Eine elektronen-
    mikroskopische Untersuchung. Beitr.Path. Bd. 157:
    340-366, 1976.

5. THE PATHOLOGY OF PARANEOPLASTIC ENCEPHALOMYELOPATHIES

D. Moffie, S.Z. Stefanko

Paraneoplastic disorders may be defined as diseases which are due to tumours elsewhere in the body but not caused by a local metastasis or tumour infiltrations. Other terms used in literature are paracarcinomatous syndrome and meta-carcinomatous syndrome.

Some tumours may have para- or metaneoplastic endocrine and metabolic effects for instance:

m. Cushing- in the oat-cell type of bronchial carcinoma,

polycythaemia- in haemangioblastoma and in hypernephroma,

acanthosis nigricans - in carcinoma of the stomach,

dermatomyositis - in bronchial carcinoma,

amyloidosis - in plasmocytoma,

porphyria - in adenoma of the liver, bronchial oat-cell
	carcinoma, adeno-carcinoma of the colon,

myasthaenia gravis - in thymona,

microthromboses - in carcinoma of the stomach and in carci-
	noma of the pancreas,

hyperadrenalism - in adrenal tumours,

hypercalcaemia - in adenoma of the parathyreoid etc.

All these effects may lead to neurological symptoms which are however out of the scope of this survey.

Our theme are the neurological paraneoplastic syndromes in the more restricted sense: the encephalomyelopathies.

This is a typical multidisciplinair subject. Though up till now most of the publications have come from clinical neurology, a lesser number from neuropathology and general pathology. In this paper we will restrict ourselves to neuropathology and to some comments as to the hypothesis

concerning etiology and pathogenesis of these enigmatic
diseases.

In the neuropathological files of our institute covering the years 1965-1979, we found 41 cases with neuropathological abnormalities in tumours elsewhere in the body
(without infiltrations in the central nervous system or metastases to the central nervous system). The age of the patients was between 40 and 80 years, the average age being
60 years. The sex ratio was equal: 21 males and 20 females.
29 Patients were in the age group of 50-70 years, 12 patients were below 50 and above 70 years. In 16 cases the
primary carcinoma was in the lung. From these 14 were males and 2 females. 5 Patients had cancer of the stomach,
5 patients (females) had breastcancer and 4 patients cancer
of the oesophagus. There were 9 patients with a primary
carcinoma in different organs: pancreas, ovary, os sacrum,
galbladder, colon, prostate, larynx, liver and kidney. In
two cases no primary tumour could be found, although metastases outside the central nervous system were present. From
these series we have selected 23 well documented cases with
striking clinical symptoms and definite neuropathological
abnormalities.

The paracarcinomatous disorders may be subdivided, as
is done in literature into the following groups:

I progressive multifocal leukoencephalopathy (PML).
II Encephalomyelitis: a. *limbic encephalitis*,
                       b. *brain stem encephalitis*,
                       c. *poliomyelitis, radiculitis,
                          neuritis.*
III Subacute cerebellar degeneration.

This subdivision, as most in medicine, is artificial.
Some groups overlap and in others there are difficulties in
classification.

I. Progressive multifocal leukoencephalopathy (PML).

PML has a somewhat separate place in the paraneoplastic
disorders. It occurs mostly in Hodgkin disease and in the
non-Hodgkin lymphomas. From the clinical point of view this

disease is characterized by subacute progressive mental
deterioration with amnesia and diffuse disturbances in the
E.E.G. Macroscopic examination of the brain is mostly negative but microscopy reveals extensive multifocal destruction of the white matter of the hemispheres; the foci are
irregular and sharply delimited. The brain stem and cerebellum are usually spared as well as the cortex of the
hemispheres and the U-fibres.

In our series only one patient with PML could be found.
This patient, a male, had a fungous carcinoma of the
stomach which was found accidentally at autopsy. For the
last 6 months of his life this 76 year old patient stayed
in a psychiatric institute on account of mental deterioration. The cause of death was bronchopneumonia. Microscopy
of the brain revealed multifocal demyelination of the white
matter in both hemispheres with irregular but sharply delimited borders (Figs. 1 and 2).

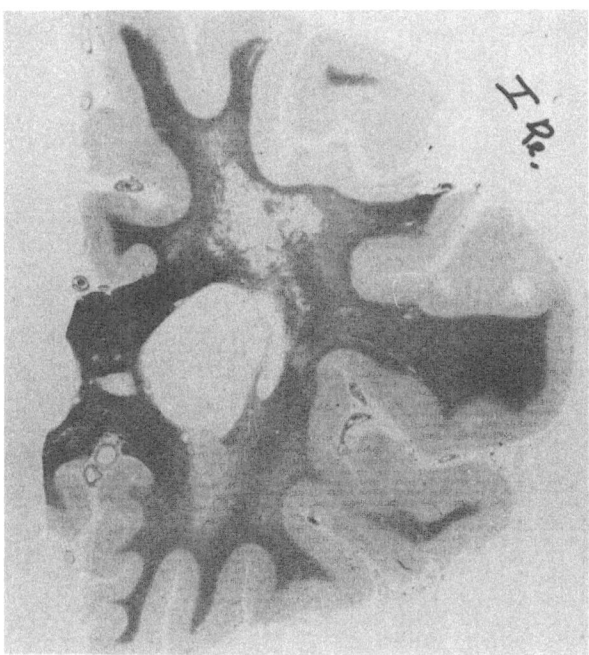

Figure 1: Progressive multifocal
leukoencephalopathy (PML).
Confluent demyelinisation of the
centrum semiovale. Klüver stain.

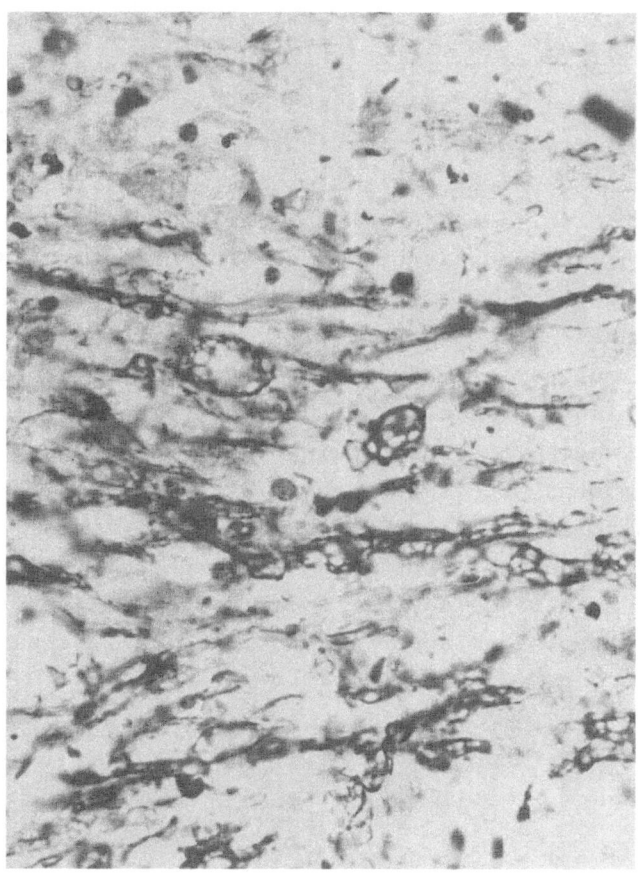

Figure 2: PML. Area of myelin destruction with ellipsoids. x 600.
Klüver stain.

The lesions were localized in the frontal-parietal and occipital areas, especially in the right parieto-occipital
region. There was a remarkable glial reaction in the areas
of demyelination with an excessive proliferation of bizarre
giant, multi-nucleated gemistocytic astrocytes, with hyper-
chromatic nuclei (fig. 3). Deeply staining homogenous
nuclei of oligodendrocytes were also seen.

Comment

This was our only case of PML and, as mentioned, primary
carcinoma of the stomach was found. In our series of 20
primary lymphomas of the brain and in the group of extra-
cerebral lymphomas (Hodgkin included) no cases of PLM
were found.

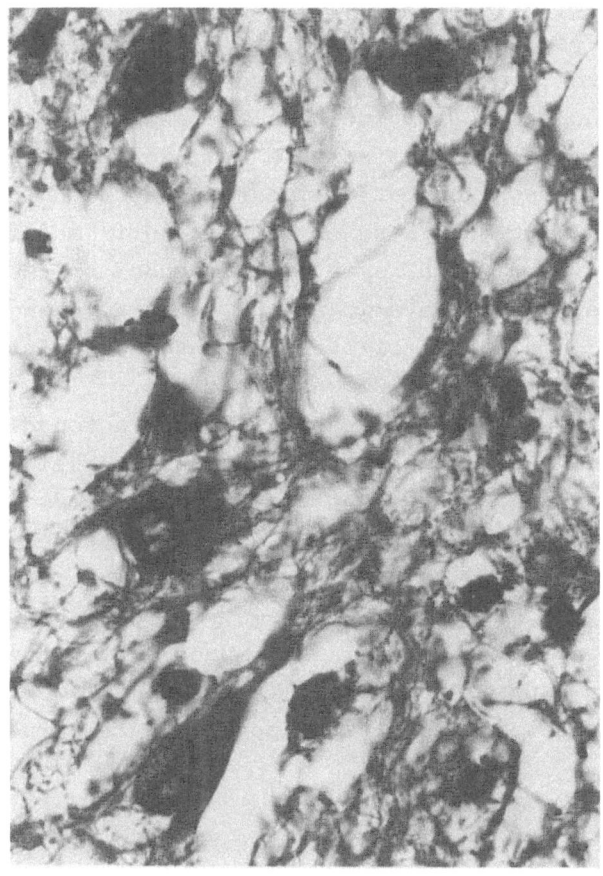

Figure 3: PML. Giant astrocytes
in the demyelinated areas.
x 600. H.E. stain.

Uptill some years ago PML has been considered as a paraneoplastic disease but the real pathogenesis was unknown. In
some cases virus particles (paramyxovirus-like structures)
have been found (ZuRhein, 1972). This has led to the view
that PML is due to a combined infection by papova and para-
myxovirus in people with a long lasting immunological sup-
pression. In our case immunosuppressive therapy had not
been used, the carcinoma was an accidental finding and no
inclusion bodies were seen. Though the microscopic picture
and the localization were typical, it was difficult to
establish a relation between the PML and the carcinoma of
the stomach.

II. Encephalomyelitis

a. *Limbic encephalitis.*

There were three cases of limbic encephalitis; one was combined with brain stem encephalitis and one case combined with polomyelitis, radiculitis and neuritis. The patients were suffering from oat-cell carcinoma of the lung. In one case the lungtumour was very small and it was found only at autopsy. The clinical symptoms, depended on the localization were: mental deterioration, amnesia, changes of personality, disturbances of conciousness and confusional states and epilepsy. The E.E.G. was aspecific.

The most striking abnormalities are found in the limbic system, which comprises the gyrus cinguli, hippocampal gyrus, fascia dentata, nucleus amygdalae, mamillary bodies, fornix and the medial part of the third temporal gyrus.

In the first case (63 year old man) perivascular lymphocytic infiltrations were seen, especially in the hippocampus (sector of Sommer), accompanied by circulatory disturbances (spongionecrosis). There were also microglial nodules and neuronal degeneration with satellitosis and neuronophagia.

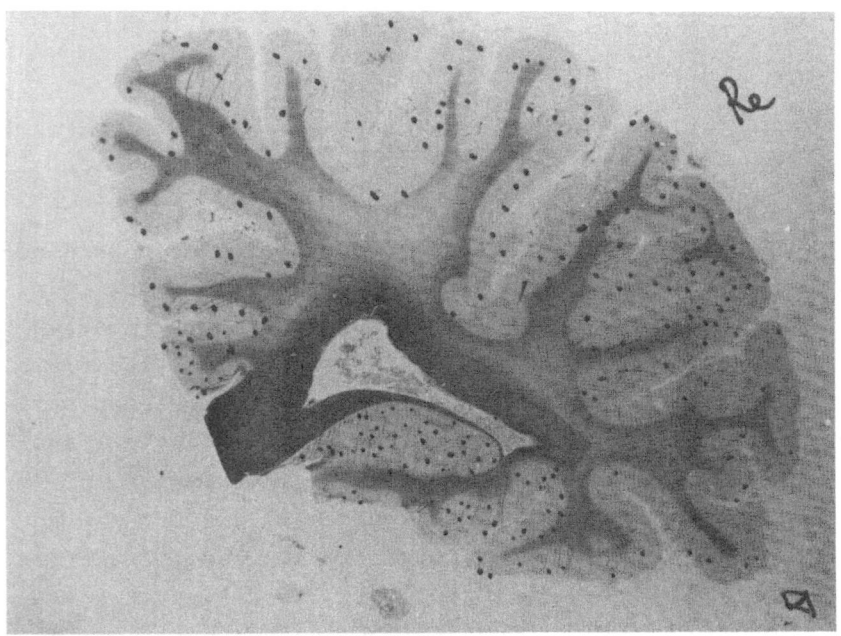

Fig. 4: see description Figure 5.

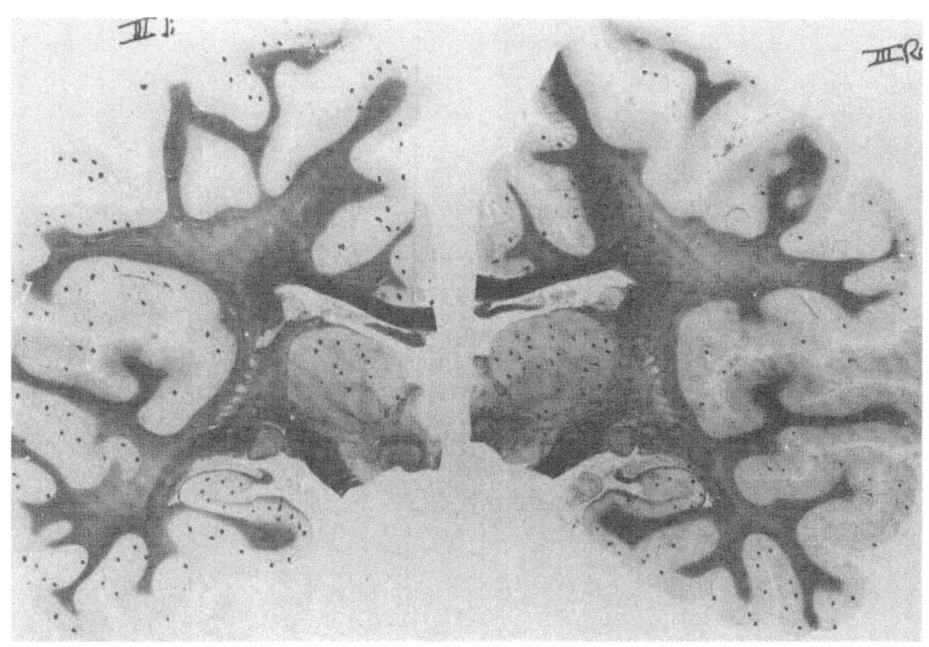

Figures 4 and 5: Limbic encephalitis (case 2). The topography of the lesions is marked by dots. Note the predilection of the lesions to the gray matter, especially to the limbic areas. Klüver stain.

In the second patient, 70 year old male, inflammatory changes were observed also in the hemispheres (Figs. 4 and 5), in the brain stem and in the spinal cord. The changes were restricted to the gray matter, the white matter not being affected. The most intensive perivascular infiltrations and glial nodules (figs. 6,7,8 and 9) were found in the nucleus amygdalae, hippocampus, hypothalamus and to a much lesser degree in other areas of the gray matter. The perivascular lymphocytic cuffs were also seen in the dorsal part of the pons and of the medulla oblongata. No infiltrations were observed in the cerebellum but there was an evidence of microglial proliferation in the molecular layer. In the gray matter of the spinal cord some infiltrations were seen in all levels, combined with focal proliferation

62

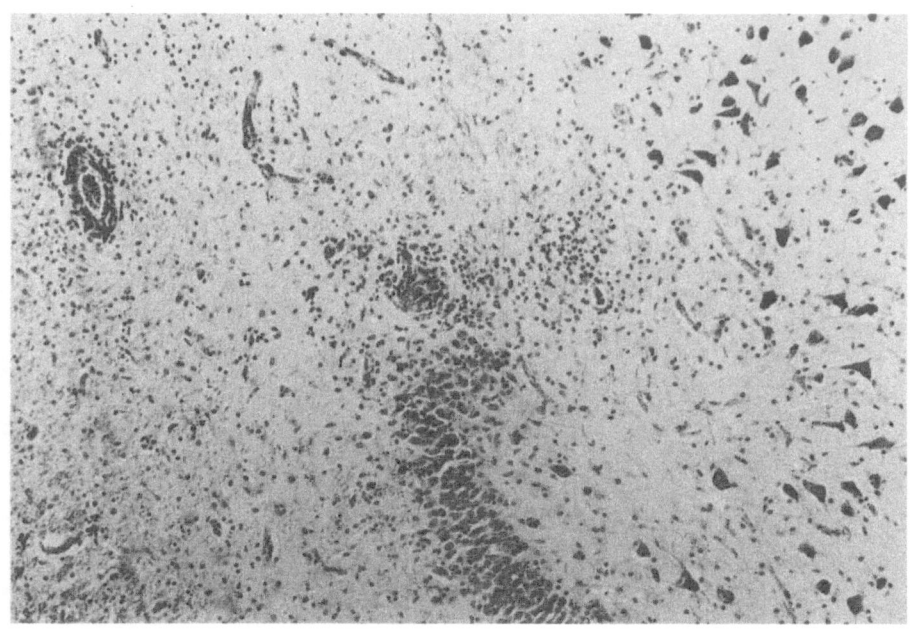

Figure 6: Limbic encephalitis. Hippocampal area.
Perivascular infiltrations and glial nodules. x 150,
Klüver stain.

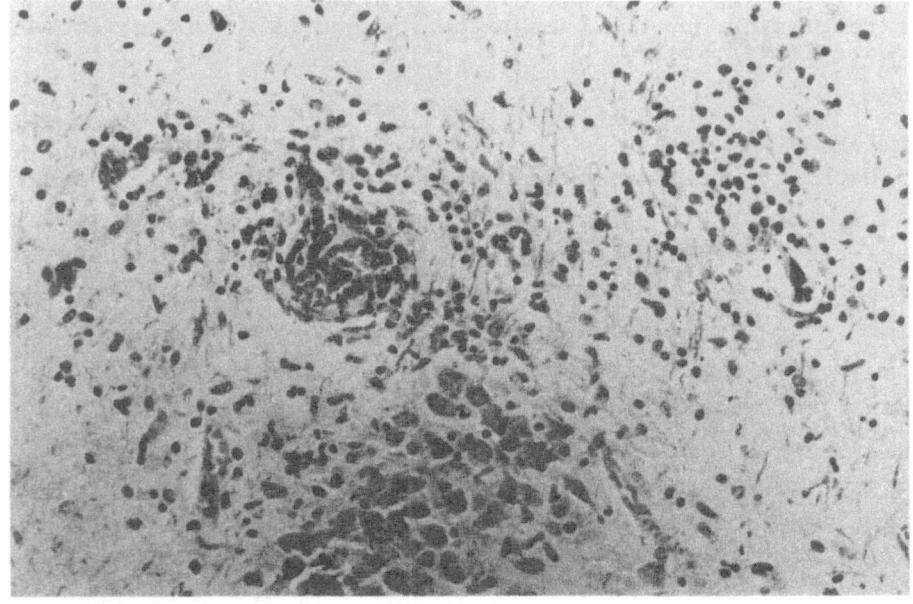

Figure 7: Detail from Figure 5. x 380, Klüver stain.

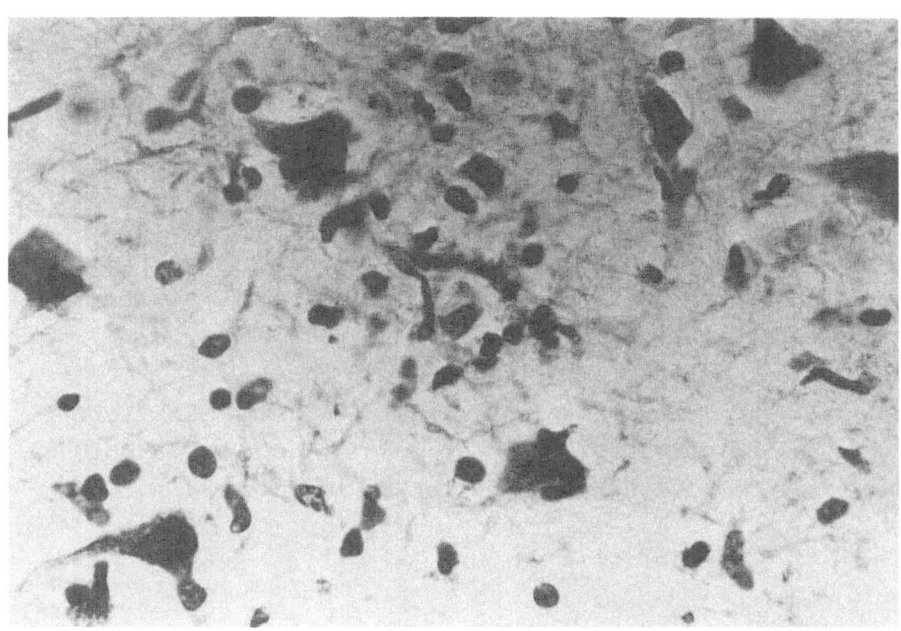

Figure 8: Limbic encephalitis. Microglial nodule. x 600,
Klüver stain.

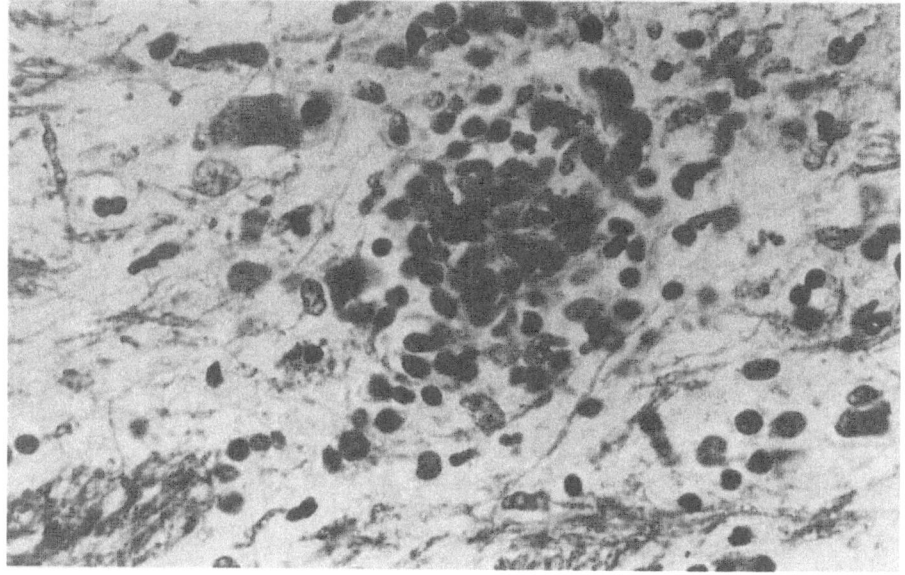

Figure 9: Limbic encephalitis. Neuronophagia. x 600,
Klüver stain.

of microglia. In this case a tentative diagnosis of paracarcinomatous encephalopathy was made before death.

In a third patient (male, 58 years old) diffuse glial
activity was seen with mild perivascular lymphocytic
reaction in the limbic areas, accompanied by a mild lymphocytic infiltration of the meninges.

b. *Bulbar and brain-stem encephalitis.*
One case of bulbar encephalitis was seen in a 69 year old
man with the symptoms of bulbar paralysis, dysarthria, paresis and atrophy of the tongue, dysphagia and vomiting;
further an external ophtalmoplegia, nystagmus, ataxia, myoclonus, and extrapyramidal symptoms.

Microscopic examinations revealed perivascular infiltrations and an microglial reaction in the medulla oblongata (fig. 10), in the pons and in the mesencephalon.

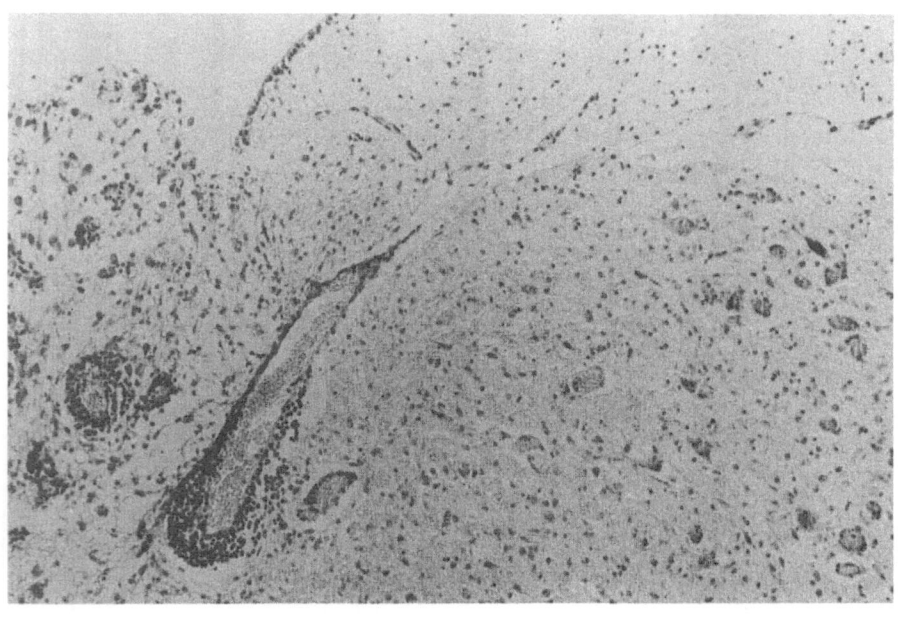

Figure 10: Bulbar encephalitis.
Medulla oblongata. Mononuclears
cuffing the small intracerebral
veins. x 150. Klüver stain.

c. *Poliomyelitis*.

One case of poliomyelitis was seen in a 60 year old man. During the clinical observation polyneuropathy on the base of malignancy and vitamin deficiency was suspected. A diagnosis of paraneoplastic amyotrophic lateral sclerosis had also been considered. On general autopsy a small oat-cell carcinoma of the left main bronchus was found with metastases in the regional lymphnodes.

On microscopic examination of the central nervous system the lesions were restricted to the spinal cord, nerve roots and peripheral nerves (fig. 11). From a pure pathological point of view it was the picture of a poliomyelitis anterior combined with radiculitis and neuritis.

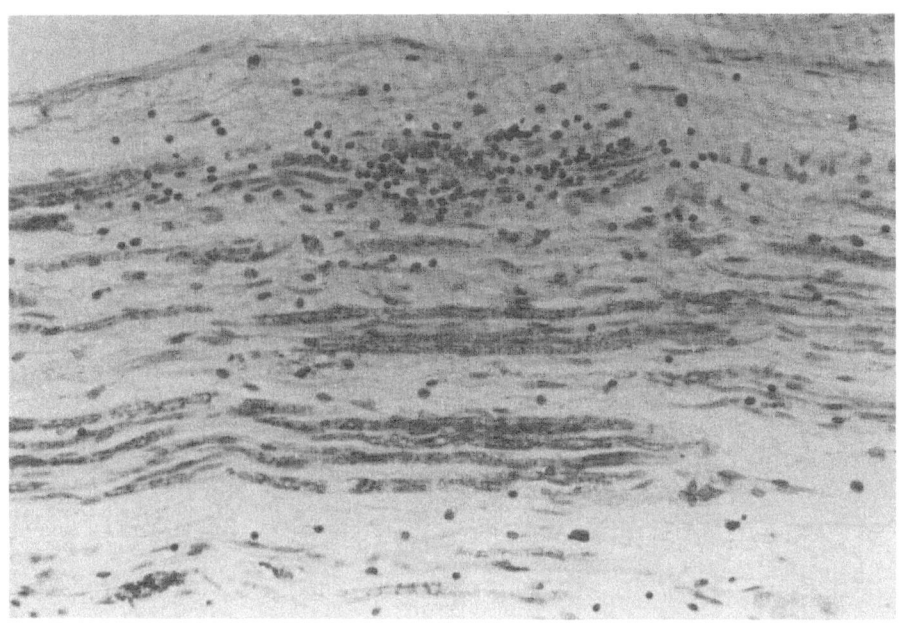

Figure 11: Paraneoplastic neuritis.
Sural nerve. Mononuclear infiltrations
and segmental degeneration of the myelin.
x 380. Klüver stain.

III. Subacute cerebellar degeneration

This was the most frequent type of paracarcinomatous encephalopathy in our series. It had a subacute course (2 - 3
months), as compared to the chronic course of the systemic
cerebellar atrophies. In our series 15 cases of this complication were found. In 6 of them the primary tumour was
a bronchial carcinoma. In two cases a carcinoma of the
oesophagus was found and in the rest of the cases carcinomas of mamma, ovary, larynx, sarcoma of the sacrum and
leukemia. In two of the cases no primary tumour could be
found although multiple metastases were present.

Cerebellar signs are predominant in the clinical picture. The most typical neuropathological abnormality was diffuse loss of Purkinje-cells (fig. 12) with normal Golgi-
cells, which formed the so-called empty baskets (fig. 13).

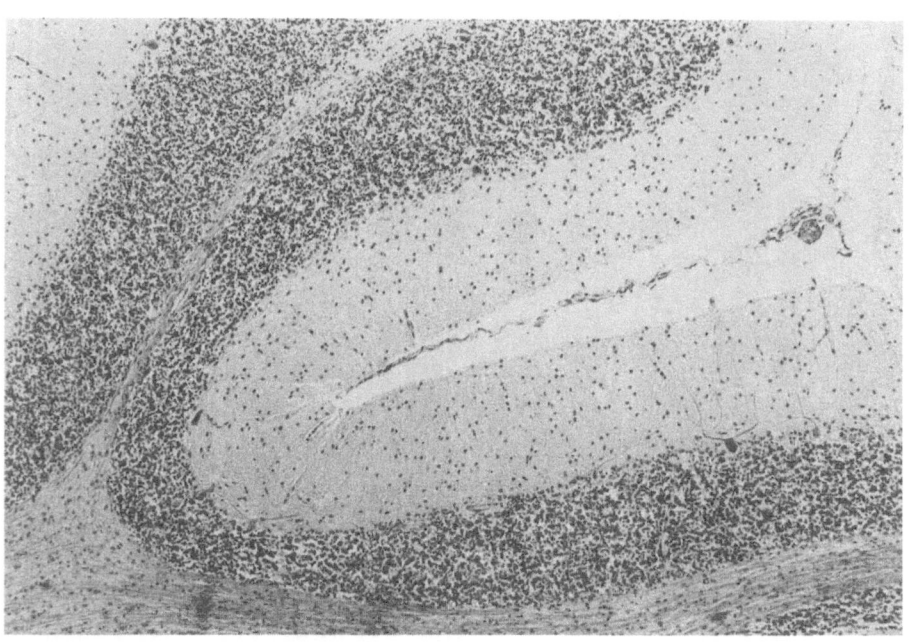

Figure 12: Subacute degeneration
of the cerebellum. Elective loss
of Purkinje-cells.
x 60. Klüver stain.

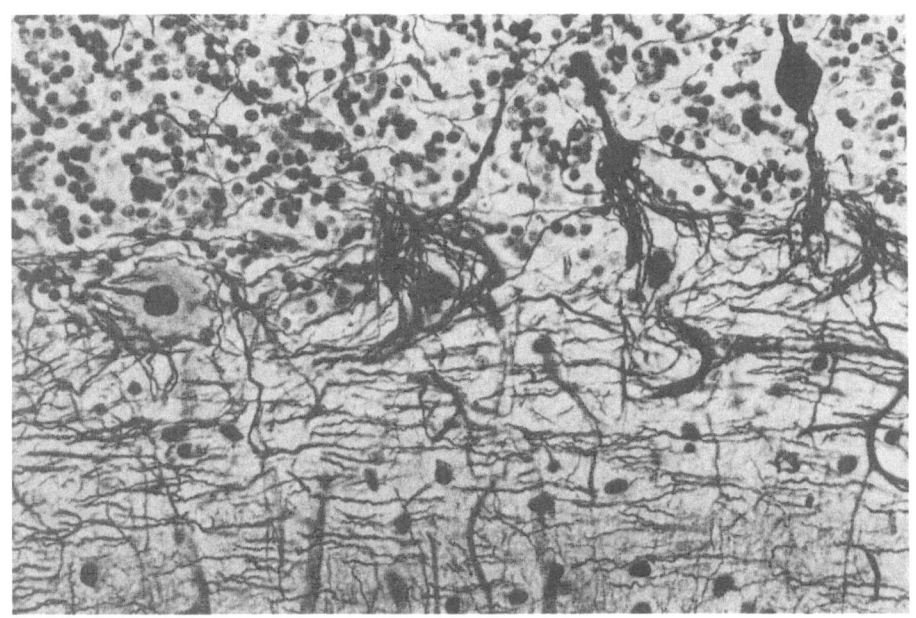

Figure 13: Disappearance of Purkinje-
cell with empty baskets and torpedos.
x 600. Bodian stain.

Furthermore proliferation of the Bergman glia was seen.
Contrasting with other cerebellar atrophies, no abnormalities in the inferior olives, dentate nucleus and in the
pons were observed. In one case necrosis of the granular
zone occurred and in one case inflammatory infiltrations
were noted.

Wernicke type encephalopathy was found in three cases.
In one of these there was also a degeneration of the posterior columns and of the pyramidal tracts. One case was
combined with neuropathy.

Comment

Paracarcinomatous encephalitis and myelitis occurs only in
a small percentage of malignant tumours which is mostly an
oat-cell carcinoma of the lung. Especially in limbic encephalitis the primary lungtumour may be very small and it is

often only found after close examination during autopsy.
Limbic encephalitis was first described by Brierley et al.
(1960) under the name "subacute encephalitis of the adult
life, mainly affecting the limbic areas". This limbic encephalitis is only a specific localization of an encephalomyelitis (Henson et al. 1965) which also comprises bulbar
encephalitis, myelitis and ganglioradiculitis. In one case
of Henson et al. (1965)(patient with oat-cell carcinoma of
the lung) lesions were scattered throughout the whole central nervous system. A more limited limbic encephalitis has
been seen by Glaser and Pinkus (1969) in 5 patients. In one
of these was an oat-cell carcinoma of the bronchus.
Corsellis et al. (1968) described three cases and stressed
the motion of "limbic encephalitis" as an entity in connection with a carcinoma. These publications have been followed by other papers which pointed to the remarkable co-
incedence between oat-cell carcinoma of the lung and encephalitis or encephalomyelitis. For a recent review of the
literature we refer to the chapters of Norris, Bruin, and
of Henson and Urich in volume 38 of the Handbook of Clinical Neruolgy (1979).

Is the coincidence between cancer and disorders of the
nervous system accidentally, by chance, or is there some
pathogenetic relation ?

There are quite a lot of theories but none has been
proven. One may ask oneself if there exists a specific relation, as the same disorders have also been described
without a malignant tumour (Wilner and Brody, 1968). In our
view the following points are important for the analysis of
these disorders.

The structure of the neuropathological process is identical with that of the known viral encephalitis respectively myelitis which consists of the triad:

a. perivascular cuffs of mononuclear cells (what we
   call inflammatory infiltration does not always mean
   infection),
b. glial nodules (reaction of the microglia) and
c. neurotropism (lesions of neurons with glial satellitosis and neuronophagia).

The limbic localization is well known and pathognomonic in herpes simplex encephalitis; but there is an important difference in the character of the lesions. In herpes simplex encephalitis there is a pronounced heamorrhagic necrotic component (acute necrotizing encephalitis) which may be easily seen on macroscopic inspection of the brain; paracarcinomatous limbic encephalitis is only detected microscopically.

Dayan, Bhatti and Gostling (1967) isolated the herpes simplex virus from the temporal lobe of a 63 year old woman who died of acute panencephalitis ("soon after she had been treated for the carcinoma of the uterus"). Dayan et al. suggest that the tumour depressed the immunity of this patient, in such a way, that the infection by herpes simplex had an unusual effect; it didnot cause the typical herpes encephalitis.

In this stage of our knowledge it is premature to equate limbic encephalitis with herpes simplex infection. To stress again: inflammation doesnot always mean infection.

In the group with localization in the brain stem and in the spinal cord, the structure of the process and its topography, strongly resembled the neuropathological picture of some viral infections, e.g. poliomyelitis. But besides these abnormalities, there are also well known other, pure degenerative changes in the spinal cord, for instance subacute necrotic myelopathy (Hoffman, 1955), without inflammation and microglial nodules. Different degenerative and inflammatory processes may overlap each other, hampering analysis.

The crucial point of this subject remains the relation: tumour-neurological symptoms (and their morphological equivalents). Often the tumour is very small and is only found at autopsy. In limbic encephalitis the survival may last up till two years. If encephalitis is indeed "related to" the carcinoma, why do these patients live so long and why is the tumour process so limited ? The life expectancy in patients with oat-cell carcinoma is much shorter (about 6 - 8 months). Why in some cases the process remains restricted to the regional lymphnodes and why there is sometimes no tendency at all to metastasing ?

Shapiro (1976) has the following explanation !

The same processes, which lead to retardation of the growth of the tumour and to the limitation of the tumoral process, modify the reactivity of neural tissue. So patients with paracarcinomatous symptoms represent a selected group with unknown defence mechanisms, which prolong survival, but on the other hand lead to characteristic reactions of the central nervous system.

There are more arguments which support the idea of an immunolgical mechanism : there is an "antigenic simularity" between the brain and the T-lymphocytes (Birnbaum,1975), between oat-cells and brain (respectively between oat-cells and lymphocytes)(Shapiro, 1976). Successfull defense against the tumour causes that the tumour remains small and limited, prolonging survival of the patient. At the same time there is more chance for the occurrence of paracarcinomatous complications which eventually lead to death.

The pathomechanism of the Wernicke-type lesions which have also been seen in some cases of subacute cerebellar degeneration are difficult to explain. In the first place we think of a relation with metabolic diseases, vitamin deficiency (as in chronic alcoholism), chronic infectious diseases and cachexia. However, in paracarcinomatous cerebellar degenerations no clear deficiencies have been found.

Aspecific causes as for instance anoxia are also to be considered. It is known that Purkinje-cells are very susceptible to anoxia. From Schenk and Enters' investigations (1970) in counting the number of Purkinje-cells in different ages became clear, that there is a progressive decrease of Purkinje-cells in later life.

Wilner and Brody (1968) compared the clinical signs of a group of 106 patients with lungcarcinoma with a control group of 44 patients without a lung tumour. They came to the conclusion, that the neurological symptoms are more related to the condition of the patients, than to the carcinoma. They thought that most of the remote effect of carcinoma are caused by aspecific nutritional deficiences and by endocrinological, immunological or metabolic abnormalities. These occur in different chronic diseases of the lungs,

including carcinoma. It has to be mentioned that the observations of Wilner and Brody were purely clinical without
anatomical verification.

CONCLUSION
The paraneoplastic encephalopathies form a heterogenic
group. Besides the progressive multifocal leukoencephalopathy (in which the viral genesis seems to be proven), the
other paraneoplastic disorders (i.e.: limbic encephalitis,
bulbar and brain-stem encephalitis, myelitis, subacute cerebellar degeneration and Wernicke-like encephalopathy) remain pathogenetically an enigma. Immunological mechanisms
seem to be an important factor in these disorders.

REFERENCES

1. Birnbaum, G, Studies on brain-thymus cross-reactive antigens. Brain Res. 84: 111-121, 1975.
2. Brierley, JB, Corsellis, JAN, Hierons, R, Nevin,S, Subacute encephalitis of later adult life mainly affecting the limbic areas. Brain, 83: 357-368, 1960.
3. Bruyn, GW, Carcinomatous polyneuropathy, In: Handbook of Clinical Neurology, Vinken, PJ, Bruyn, GW (eds.), North Holland Publ.Corp. 38: 669-677, 1979.
4. Corsellis, JAN, Goldberg, GJ, Norton, AR,"Limbic encephalitis" and its association with carcinoma. Brain, 91: 481-496, 1968.
5. Dayàn , AD, Bhatti, I, Gostling JVT. cit. in: Corsellis et al. 1968.
6. Glaser, GH, Pinkus, JH, Limbic encephalitis. J.Nerv.Ment.Dis. 149: 59-67, 1969.
7. Henson, RA, Hoffman, HL, Urich, H, Encephalomyelitis with carcinoma. Brain, 88: 449-464, 1965.
8. Henson, RA, Urich, H, Remote effects of malignant disease: certain intracranial disorders. In:Handbook of Clinical Neurology , Vinken, PJ, Bruyn, GW (eds.) North Holland Publ.Corp. 38: 625-668, 1979.

9.   Hoffman, HL, Acute necrotic myelopathy. Brain, 78: 377-393, 1955.

10.   Norris Jr., FH, Remote effects of cancer on the spinal cord. In: Handbook of Clinical Neurology, Vinken,PJ, Bruyn,GW (eds.) North Holland Publ.Corp. 38:669-677, 1979.

11.   Shapiro, WR, Remote effects of neoplasm on the Central Nervous System: Encephalopathy. In: Advances in Neurology, Thompson, RA, Green, JR (eds.) Raven Press, New York, 15: 101-117, 1976.

12.   Schenk, VWD, Enters, JH, Evaluation of Purkinje cell Density. Psychiatria Neurologica Neurochirurgia, 73: 77-86, 1970.

13.   Wilner,EC, Brody, JA, An evaluation of the remote effects of cancer on the nervous system. Neurology, 18: 1120-1124, 1968.

14.   ZuRhein, GM, Virions in progressive multifocal leukencephalopathy. In: Pathology of the Nervous System. Minckler, J,(Ed.) McGraw-Hill Book Company, 3: 2893-2912, 1972.

6. TREATMENT OF BRAIN AND SPINAL METASTASES

J. Hildebrand

A prospective study of the distribution of neurological lesions seen
during a 5 year-period in 696 consecutive patients admitted to the
Institut Jules Bordet, Brussels, a general cancer hospital, indicated
that almost 75% of these disorders are due to metastases or to local
extension of the tumor (1). Among them, brain metastases figure pro-
minently accounting for over 30% of all neurological diseases seen in
these cancer patients, whereas spinal metastases are approximately 5
times less frequent.
Both conditions are severe and life threatening. Their treatment
constitutes a major and difficult challange. Special efforts have been
recently directed to prevent or at least, to lower the incidence of
these complications. Therefore, in this review, a distinction will be
made between the so called prophylactic treatment which aims to erra-
dicate the undetected and often undetectable secondary neoplastic
deposits from treatments of clinically appearent metastatic lesions of
the nervous system.

PROPHYLACTIC TREATMENT OF BRAIN METASTASES

In patients with solid tumors, prophylactic treatment of brain metastases has been advocated and is still used in patients with small cell

anaplastic carcinoma (oat cell carcinoma). The reasons for this prophylaxis are :
a) the high incidence of brain metastases in oat cell carcinoma (2)
b) the fairly good sensitivity of this tumor to irradiations
c) the prolongation of life of these patients by combination of drugs
   poorly crossing the blood-brain barrier and leaving the brain unprotected for the development of secondary tumors. Thus, brain
   metastases appear theoretically as a major factor limiting further
   therapeutic progress in this disease.

The prophylactic treatment of brain metastases in patients with oat
cell carcinoma of the lung consists of irradiation of the whole brain,
the most current dose being 3000 rads given in 10 to 14 fractions. In
the first trials using prophylactic brain irradiation, the effect of
this treatment on the incidence of brain metastases was not quantitati-
vely evaluated nor did these studies contain non-irradiated controls
(3,4). The first two controlled studies (5,6) have demonstrated a
significant decrease in the incidence of brain metastases in patients
treated by cranial irradiation (table 1) but no significant increase
in the survival. In the largest of the two studies (6) the benefit of
the prophylactic brain irradiation was found only in patients who did
not achieve a complete remission (table 1). This observation is somewhat conflicting with the data published by Levitt et al (7) where,
despite cranial irradiation, brain metastases were found only in
patients with partial remission (table 1).
The decrease in cerebral metastases by prophylactic irradiation with
2,000 rads was not demonstrated by Cox et al (8) in patients with oat
cell carcinoma. However, the irradiation was sufficient to reduce or
delay the appearance of brain metastases in patients with squamous
large cell and adenocarcinoma of the lung.

Finally, a recent study by Hirsch et al (9) does not confirm the
earlier results indicating that cranial irradiation decreases the
incidence of brain metastases in patients with small cell anaplastic
carcinoma of the lung (table 1).

In conclusion, prophylactic cranial irradiation does not seem to prolong the life of patients with oat cell carcinoma. It possibly decreases the incidence of brain metastases but this has not been unequivocal
ly established. One study (8) suggests that in other types of lung
cancer, the prophylactic irradiation of the cranium may increase the
delay in the development of brain metastases.

TREATMENT OF SYMPTOMATIC BRAIN METASTASES

The choice of the best treatment, in the various clinical situations
where brain metastases are seen, remains difficult despite the large
number of studies devoted to the subject. This is due mainly to the
lack of adequately controlled trials. In addition, the duration and
the quality of the survival, often chosen as criteria for the evaluation of treatments of brain metastases are not related to brain metastases only in patients with disseminated disease. Another frequently
used criterion for treatment evaluation is objective remission. This
parameter is of course directly related to the effect of a given therapy on brain metastases, but is difficult to measure with accuracy.
The clinical improvement of patients with brain metastases is often
due to corticosteroids which act primarily on brain oedema surrounding
the tumor. In a vast majority of the studies, this effect is not clearly dissociated from those of specifically antineoplastic treatments.
Brain CT-scan possibly allows such a distinction but only rare and
recent studies include this examination.

NEUROSURGERY

Several reports indicate that surgical removal of brain metastases is
superior to no treatment. However, these retrospective and non-randomized studies are probably biased by the selection for neurosurgery of
the patients with the best prognosis. Probably the strongest argument

in favor of surgical removal of brain metastases is the rate of long
survivals observed in series of operated patients. Störtebecker (10)
operated on 125 patients and reported that 21.6% were alive one year
after operation, one patient with hypernephroma survived 17 years. In
a small series of 16 patients operated by Perese (11), 3 (18.8%) were
alive after 2 1/2 years. Even more encouraging results were obtained
by Furlow (12), 16.2% of 37 patients were alive at 6 years. Lang and
Slater (13) operated on 208 patients with brain metastases. Excluding
those with positive chest X-rays, they observed a 35% survival at 1
year, 15% at 3 years and 10% were still alive at 5 years. Out of 155
cases operated by Vieth and Odom (14), 21 (13.5%) survived the operation by one year and 6 were still living for more than 3 1/2 to 10
years. More recently, Raskind et al (15) reported in 51 operated
patients, a 30% survival one year after neurosurgery; 8% were still
alive after three years.

Reviewing retrospectively 200 patients treated at the Institut Jules
Bordet for brain metastases, we have found that only 15% survived 1
year of those 9% were operated.
Adequate (i.e. randomized) controls were used in none of these studies
and it is likely that the patients chosen for neurosurgery were those
with the best prognosis. Nevertheless, it is reasonable to assume that
exceptionally long survivals are due to the surgical removal of the
secondary tumor. However, the benefit provided by neurosurgery to a
restricted number of patients is balanced by the high rate of early
mortality which was superior to 25 and even 50% in several studies
(10, 11, 16, 17). Therefore, the question is not so much to know whether
one should or should not operate on patients with cerebral metastases
but rather how to select the cases for neurosurgery. Obviously, postoperative mortality may be reduced to acceptable figures such as 5.4%
by adequate patient selection (12). Although it is not possible to
establish rigid eligibility rules for neurosurgery in patients with
brain metastases, several criteria emerge from most studies :
1) Patients must be in good general condition and have a minimal extra-
   neural neoplastic burden;
2) In case of favorable neurosurgical outcome, the expected survival
   should be superior to 6 months;

3) Brain metastases must appear unique after a careful investigation and should appear totally removable, since biopsies and partial resections are accompanied by an increased rate of early deaths;

4) Slowly growing tumors, those which have a long interval between the diagnosis of the primary neoplasm and the control metastases probably have a better post-neurosurgical prognosis. These tumors, however, include hypernephroma, thyroid carcinomas or testicular tumors which account, unfortunately, for a small percentage of primaries in brain metastases.

RADIOTHERAPY

Radiotherapy appears today essentially as a prophylactic treatment; its goal is to prolong and improve the quality of the survival.
The improvement of life quality may be achieved through partial or total regressions of the neurological symptoms and signs. Such remissions have been observed in 37 to 80% of patients (table 2) treated mainly, but not exclusively, with radiotherapy   (2,18,19,20,21,22,23). These rates of objective remissions, although very high, are not superior to those obtained with corticosteroids, which were given to most of the patients studied in these trials. In addition, a similar rate of objective remissions was found by Horton et al (24) in a randomized and prospective study where patients were treated either by Prednisone (40mg per day during four weeks) or by a combination of radiotherapy and Prednisone. However, the duration of the remission tended to be longer in irradiated patients. The fact that the initial improvement in patients irradiated for brain metastases may be due primarily to the administration of steroids, which act on the peritumoral brain oedema and which activity is not related to tumor pathology, is further consistent with the rather surprising observation (18,19) that the rate of objective remissions to irradiations is not related to the nature of the primary tumor. In another study (18) patients with squamous cell bronchogenic carcinomas did even better than those with a much more radiosensitive oat-cell tumor.

What is the best radiotherapy schedule? There is a large agreement
that the whole cranium should be irradiated because in the majority of
the cases, the metastases are multiple and disseminated. But the doses
and the time of irradiation are not standardized. By comparing the results from different centers, it would appear that in terms of rates of
objective remission and duration of survival time, similar results are
obtained by different treatments ranging from 1,000 rads given in one
dose to 4,500 rads delivered in four weeks. But, as indicated above,
those evaluation criteria are open to criticism when steroids are used.

One thousand rads given as a single dose increase the rate of complications, at least in patients with intracranial hypertension (25). From
large prospective studies, now in progress, it will probably emerge
that the administration of 3,000 rads in a 12 day-period combines safe-
ty and best efficacy.

CORTICOSTEROIDS AND CHEMOTHERAPY

Corticosteroids reduce the peritumoral cerebral oedema with regularity
and thereby improve the neurological functions, usually within 24 to
48 hours, in the majority of patients with brain metastases. The total
daily doses vary from 10 to 16mg, but higher amounts may, in some cases
improve the therapeutic results. The clinical effects of corticosteroids
are sustained as long as their administration is maintained. However,
because of some serious side-effects such as proximal myopathy or de-
pression in the immune mechanism, unnecessary high doses of corticosteroids must be avoided during the maintenance phase.

Glycerol, given p.o. at daily doses of 1.5g/kg in four fractions, is
also effective in reducing brain oedema in patients with brain metastases (26). In cases of emergency, a perfusion with 20% mannitol reduces rapidly but temporarily the oedema of the brain.

Today the role of chemotherapy in the treatment of brain metastases appears modest and requires further evaluation. Chemotherapy agents are usually combined with radiotherapy and corticosteroids. Therefore, adequate studies testing their efficacy are scarce. Often preference is given to lipid soluble drugs crossing the blood-brain barrier. Metastases do not usually infiltrate the normal brain to an extent comparable to primary tumors, and since the barrier is not preserved in the metastatic nodules, this limitation may not be justified. In our experience (27), breast carcinoma brain metastases respond better to the combination of CCNU, vincristine and methotrexate than bronchogenic secondaries. Objective remission, defined as a clinical improvement present 6 weeks after complete discontinuation of steroids and lasting 4 weeks or more was observed in 4 of 8 patients with breast cancer but only in one of 15 cases with lung carcinoma.

A similar difference between the response of breast and lung cerebral metastases was also reported by Pouillart et al (28) using the combination of VM-26 and CCNU.

TREATMENT OF EPIDURAL METASTASES

PROPHYLACTIC TREATMENT

Prophylaxis of spinal cord compression by epidural metastases per se is not a standard procedure.

However, treatment of patients with Hodgkin's disease includes, in stages I, II and IIIa, irradiation of cervical, mediastinal and lombo-aortic areas. A similar treatment is also given to patients with non-Hodgkin's lymphomas in stages I and II. Thus, in all these patients, the epidural space is irradiated totally or partially with approximately 3,000 to 4,500 rads. Since lymphomas do not usually relapse in irradiated areas, one may consider these irradiations as prophylactic treatments of epidural space metastases. We do not have figures proving the efficacy of this prophylaxis but it is reasonable to assume that the extremely low percentage (0.1%) of spinal cord compressions observed, for instance by the South-West Oncology Group in 1,039 cases of non-Hodgkin's lymphoma registered to irradiation of the spinal cord area.

In patients with other solid tumors, those with vertebral metastases appear as a high risk group with respect to epidural spinal compression. Myelography performed in such patients reveals a high percentage of partial or even complete blocks (table 3, 29). We have suggested that this examination should be performed in every patient with vertebral metastases, even in the absence of signs of spinal cord compression, especially if pain is present. Lipid-soluble dye should be used for the procedure, it will allow subsequent objective evaluation of the effects of radiotherapy which should be used as a prophylactic treatment of spinal compression in cases with abnormal myelography.

TREATMENT OF SPINAL CORD COMPRESSION

A question often asked in the past and not yet definitely answered is whether laminectomy is useful. There is a wide agreement that, in lymphomas, including Hodgkin's disease, spinal cord compression should be treated by radiotherapy and chemotherapy (NH2-mustard, vincristine, procarbazine and prednisone) without laminectomy (30, 31). These patients, however, should be maintained under supervision and laminectomy may be useful if the neurological signs fail to improve or become more conspicuous.

In other solid tumors, laminectomy has been recommended as the first treatment despite a high parcentage of disappointing results (restoration of gait and sphincter functions have been achieved in only 10 to 35%) and a high rate of morbidity (32,33 ,34 , 35, 36). Recently, Gilbert et al (37) analyzed 130 consecutive cases of spinal cord compression by extradural metastases treated by radiotherapy and 105 previously reported cases treated for the same complication at the Memorial Sloan-Kettering Cancer Center. Out of 235 patients, 65 underwent surgical decompression followed by radiotherapy and 170 were treated by irradiation alone. There was no significant difference between the two groups, even when patients with various grades of weakness at the onset of treatment were considered separately. Although this study is retrospective and non-randomized, it strongly suggests that the role of laminectomy is limited even in patients with tumors poorly sensitive to irradiation.

Chemotherapy may be added to radiotherapy. The choice of the drugs is related to the nature of the primary tumor. It should be pointed out that the metastases of the epidural space are in no way protected by the bloodbrain barrier.

Administration of corticosteroids at doses similar to those used in patients with brain metastases is a current practice in some centers. It aims to reduce the possible spinal cord oedema which may be enhanced by radiations.

IN SUMMARY

a) Early detection of metastases of the epidural space by myelography is recommended to allow their treatment before the appearance of signs of spinal cord compression.

b) In patients with clinical signs of spinal cord compression, radiotherapy should be started as soon as possible. The place of neurosurgery in the management of epidural metastases remains controversial. We feel that laminectomy should be performed when :
    - the diagnosis is uncertain ;
    - the association of radiotherapy and chemotherapy cannot be given or fails to improve the neurological status rapidly.

If laminectomy is to be performed as the first treatment, the best cases appear to be those with slowly progressing neurological signs of spinal cord compression by epidural metastases originating from tumors relatively resistant to irradiation.

TABLE 1

TRIALS TESTING PROPHYLACTIC BRAIN IRRADIATION IN SMALL CELL LUNG CARCINOMA

Ref.	Number of cases	Prophylactic treatment	Frequency of metastases	P	Mean survival	P
Jackson et al. 1977	29	14 received 3000 rads in 10 fractions	0 (0 %)	0.05	9.8 months	NS
		15 controls	4 (27 %)		7.2 months	
Tulloh et al. 1977	151 out of 171	69 received 3000 rads in 10 frac.	2 (3 %)	0.01	8.7 months	NS
		82 controls	15 (17 %)		8.5 months	
	48 out of 151	22 received 3000 rads in 10 frac.	2 (9 %)	NS	NOT SPECI- FIED	
		26 controls	4 (15 %)		NOT SPECI- FIED	

Ref.	Number of cases	Prophylactic treatment	Frequency of metastases	P	Mean survival	P
Levitt et al. 1978	15	All received 3000 rads in 12 days	CR 0/8 PR 3/7	-	35 weeks	
		Same treatment	CR 0/1 PR 2/8 NR 0/5	-	23 weeks	
Cox et al. 1978	24	2000 rads in 10 fractions and 2 weeks	4 (17 %)	NS	NOT SPECI- FIED FOR PATIENTS	
	21	controls	5 (24 %)		WITH OAT- CELL CARCINOMA	
Hirsch, Hansen et al. 1979	111	55 received 4000 rads in 4 weeks	5 (9 %)	NS	310 days	NS
		56 controls	7 (13 %)		281 days	

TABLE 2

RESULTS IN RADIOTHERAPY IN THE TREATMENT OF BRAIN METASTASES

REFERENCES	N° OF EVALUABLE PATIENTS	NEUROLOGICAL IMPROVEMENT
CHAO ET AL. (1954)	38	63%
DEELEY & EDWARDS	61	47% "Significant Palliation "
ORDER ET AL. (1968)	108	60% (27% at 6 months 5% at 1 year)
NISCE ET AL. (1971)	376	80% (Mean Duration of Improvement = 5 mo.)
MONTANA ET AL. (1972)	62	56%
DEUTSCH ET AL. (1974)	88	"The Majority Improved"
NEWMAN & HANSEN (1974)	45	27% "Good Response"
SHEHATA ET AL. (1974)	81	35% Excellent Response 40% Fair Response 25% No Response

TABLE 3

MYELOGRAPHY FINDINGS IN 75 PATIENTS WITH VERTEBRAL METASTASES

Clinical Group	Number of Cases	Normal	Partial Block	Complete Block
No Neurological Symptoms	6	4	2	0
Radicular Pain No Signs of Spinal Cord Compression	52	26	15	11
Signs of Spinal Cord Compression	17	5	2	10

REFERENCES

1. Hildebrand J. (1978) : Lesions of the nervous system in cancer
    patients. Raven Press, New-York

2. Newman S.J. & Hansen H.H. (1974) : Frequency, diagnosis and treat-
    ment of brain metastases in 247 consecutive patients with broncho-
    genic carcinoma. Cancer, 33: 492-496

3. Johnson R.E., Brereton H.D. & Kent C.H. (1976) : Small-cell
    carcinoma of the lung : attempts to remedy causes of post-
    therapeutic failure. Lancet ii: 289-291

4. Livingston R.B. & Moore T.N. (1976) : Combined modality treatment
    of oat cell carcinoma of the lung. Proc. Am. Assoc. Cancer Res.
    & ASCO 17: 152

5. Jackson D.V., Richards F., Cooper R., Feree C., Muss H.B., White
    D.R. & Spurr C.L. (1977) : Prophylactic cranial irradiation in
    small cell carcinoma of the lung. A randomized study. JAMA 237:
    2730-2733

6. Tulloh M.E., Maurer L.H. & Foncier R.J. (1977) : A randomized trial
    of prophylactic whole brain irradiation in small cell carcinoma of
    the lung. Proc. Am. Soc. Clin. Oncol. 18: 268

7. Levitt M., Meikle A., Murray N. & Weinerman B. (1978) : Oat cell
    carcinoma of the lung : CNS metastases in spite of prophylactic
    brain irradiation. Cancer Treat. rapp. 62: 131-133

8. Cox J.D., Petrovich Z., Paig C. & Stanley K. (1978) : Prophylactic
    cranial irradiation in patients with inoperable carcinoma of the
    lung. Preliminary report of a cooperative trial. Cancer, 42:
    1135-1140

9. Hirsch F., Hansen H.H., Paulson A.B. & Vraa-Jensen J. : Develop-
    ment of brain metastases in small cell onaplastic carcinoma of the
    lung. In "CNS complications of malignant disease". Kay & White-
    house, ed. Ma Millan Press. 1979, pp. 175-184

10. Störtebecker T.P. (1954) : Metastatic tumors of the brain from a
    neurological point of view (a follow-up study of **158 cases**).
    J. Neurosurg., 11: 84-111

11. Perese D.M. (1959) : Prognosis in metastatic tumors of the brain
    and the skull : An analysis of 16 operative and 162 autopsied cases.
    Cancer, 12: 609-613

12. Furlow L.T. (1963) : Metastatic tumors of the brain. Clin. Neuro-
    surg., 7: 63-78

13. Lang E. & Slater J. (1964) : Metastatic brain tumors. Results of
    surgical and neurological treatment. Surg. Clin. North. Am., 44:
    865-872

14. Vieth R.G. & Odom G.L. (1965) : Intracranial metastases and their neurosurgical treatment. J. Neurosurg. 23: 375-383

15. Raskind R., Weiss S.R., Manning O. & Wermuth R.A. (1971) : Survival after surgical incision of single metastatic tumors. Amer. J. Roentgen, 3: 323-328

16. Simionescu M.E. (1960) : Metastatic tumors of the brain. A follow-up study of 195 patients with neurosurgical considerations. J. Neurosurg., 17: 361-373

17. Richars P. & McKissock W. (1963) : Intracranial metastases. Br. Med. J. 1: 15-18

18. Chao J.H., Phillips R. & Nickerson J.J. (1954) : Roentgen-ray therapy of cerebral metastases. Cancer, 7: 682-689

19. Deeley T.J. & Edwards J.M.R. (1968) : Radiotherapy in the management of cerebral secondaries from bronchial carcinoma. Lancet, 1: 1209-1212

20. Order S.E., Hellman S., Vonessen C.F. & Kligerman M.M. (1968) : Improvement in quality of survival following whole-brain irradiation for brain metastasis. Radiology, 91: 149-153

21. Nisce L.Z., Hilaris B.S. & Chu F.C.H. (1971) : A review of experience with irradiation of brain metastasis. Am. J. Roentgenol 111: 329-333

22. Montana G.S., Meacham W.F. & Caldwell W.L. (1972) : Brain irradiation for metastatic disease of lung origin. Cancer, 29: 1477-1480

23. Shehata W.M., Hendrickson F.R. & Hindo W.A. (1974) : Rapid fractionation technique and re-treatment of cerebral metastases by irradiation. Cancer, 34:257-261

24. Horton J., Baxter D.H., Olson K.B. & The Eastern Cooperative Oncology Group (1971) : The management of metastases to the brain by irradiation and corticosteroids. Am. J. Roentgenol 11:334-336

25. Posner J.B., Chu F.C.H. & Nisce L.Z. (1974) : Rapid course radiation therapy of brain metastases. ASCO Abstr. (n° 752) pp 172

26. Bedikian A.Y., Valdivieso M. & Withers H.R. (1977) : Glycerol, a new alternative to dexamethasone in patients receiving brain irradiation. Abstr. AARC, pp. 50

27. Hildebrand J., Brihaye J., Wagenknecht L., Michel J., & Kenis Y. (1973) : Combination chemotherapy with 1-(2-chloro-ethyl-3-cyclohexyl-1-nitrosourea (CCNU), vincristine and methotrexate in primary and metastatic brain tumors. A preliminary report. Europ. J. Cancer, 9: 627-634

28. Pouillart P., Mathé G., Poisson M., Buge A., Huguenin P., Gautier H., Morin P., Hoang Thy H.T., Lheritier J. & Parrot R. (1976) : Essai de traitement de glioblastomes de l'adulte et des métastases cérébrales par l'association d'adriamycine, de VM26 & de CCNU. Nouv. Presse Med. 5: 1571-1576

29. Longeval E., Hildebrand J. & Vollont G.H. (1975) : Early diagnosis of metastases in the epidural space. Acta Neurochir. 31: 177-184

30. Mullins G.M., Flynn J.P.G., El-Madhi A.M., McOreen D. & Owens A.H. Jr. (1971) : Malignant lymphoma of the spinal epidural space. Ann. Intern. Med., 74: 416-423

31. Silverberg I.J. & Jacobs E.M. (1971) : Treatment of spinal cord compression in Hodgkin's disease. Cancer, 27: 308-313

32. Wright R.L. (1963) : Malignant tumors of the spinal extradural space. Results of surgical treatment. Ann. Surg. 157: 227

33. Brice J. & McKissock W. (1965) : Surgical treatment of malignant extradural spinal tumors. Br. Med. J., 1: 1341-1344

34. Smith R.A. (1965) : An evaluation of surgical treatment for spinal cord compression due to metastatic carcinoma. J. Neurol. Neurosurg. Psychiatry, 28: 152-158

35. Vieth R.G. & Odom G.L. (1965) : Extradural spinal metastases and their neurosurgical treatment. J. Neurosurg. 23: 501-508

36. Bansal S., Brady L.W., Olsen A.O., Faust D.S., Osterholm J. & Kazem I. (1967) : The treatment of metastatic spinal cord tumors. JAMA, 202: 686-688

37. Gilbert R.W., Kim J.H. & Posner J.B. (1978) : Epidural spinal cord compression from metastatic tumor : diagnosis and treatment. Ann. Neurol. 3: 40-51.

7. THE ROLE OF RADIOTHERAPY IN THE MANAGEMENT OF INTRA-CEREBRAL METASTASES

D. Ash

INTRODUCTION

The overall incidence of cerebral metastases found at post mortem in patients dying of cancer is 15-20%. 60-70% of cases have multiple metastases in the brain and the majority are found in the cerebral hemispheres though approximately 20% may be in the cerebellum. Lung cancer and breast cancer are by far the commonest tumours which metastasise to the brain. In lung cancer the brain may be the only site of the metastasis in approximately 75% of cases whereas in breast cancer approximately 75% of cases of brain metastasis are associated with metastases elsewhere.

Although there are a few cases in which cerebral metastases are found by chance at post mortem, the majority suffer a number of distressing symptoms during their terminal illness. The commonest of these are motor disturbances, headaches, convulsions, intellectual impairment, cranial nerve abnormalities and cerebellar ataxia. These symptoms may produce varying degrees of disability which can be classified according to the System of Order et al (1968) which includes four functional classes from Class 1, which is patients with little or no neurological abnormality to Class 4 which is patients requiring hospitalisation and with severe physical and neurological disability.

If patients with cerebral metastases are untreated or given only symptomatic therapy for relief of headaches the median survival is approximately one month. There are many people who hold the view that the development of cerebral metastases is part of dying and that because of the very short survival active treatment is quite inappropriate. If, however, you believe that an attempt should be made to relieve distressing symptoms even in patients with a short survival time then, provided that treatment can achieve this, some benefit to the patient may result. Hendrickson et al (1975) have shown that cerebral radiation for metastases produces complete or partial relief of symptoms in 91% of patients having convulsions, 86% headache, 76% motor loss and 72% impaired mentation. Similar results have been reported from numerous other series and it is quite clear that radiation produces significant palliation for a large number of patients.

TREATMENT

Radiation Fields

Because of the high incidence of multiple metastases within the brain the radiation fields must encompass the entire intra-cranial contents. Occasionally smaller fields may be used to boost specific areas.

Dose/Time Factors

A very wide range of regimes for the treatment of cerebral metastases has been reported in the literature from 1000 rads in a single treatment up to 4000 rads in 20 treatments over 4 weeks. 1000 rads in a single treatment is attractive because it cuts down to a minimum the treatment time for patients with short survival. It has been noted however, (Harwood & Simpson 1977, Hindo et al 1970) that there is an increase in complication rate following single dose treatment particularly in patients with raised intra-cranial pressure at the time of treatment. A similar increase in complication rate was noted by Young et al (1973) when 1500 rads in 2 treatments was compared with 3000 rads in 15 treatments. Several fractionation studies have been performed by the Radiation Therapy Oncology Group which has reported that a dose of 3000 rads given in ten equal fractions for a two week period appeared to be the most satisfactory schedule for the majority of patients (Kramer et al 1979).

Steroid Therapy

Dexamethasone frequently produces rapid regression of neurological signs but improvement is not generally sustained for long and the side effects of prolonged treatment with Dexamethasone may themselves become disabling. Unless single or rapid course radiation is being given it is not necessary to give Dexamethasone as a routine during the course of radiation for those patients who do not have symptoms or signs of raised intra-cranial pressure.

COMPLICATIONS AND SIDE EFFECTS OF BRAIN RADIATION

Deterioration in Neurological Status

Some patients temporarily get worse during or after a course of whole brain radiation and fatal cerebral herniation has been reported particularly after rapid course treatment. It has been suggested that these complications are due to a rise in intra-cranial pressure produced by the radiation but direct measurements of CSF pressure before and after whole brain radiotherapy have shown that although elevation of pressure may occur this may not be associated with symptoms and conversely that a deterioration in symptoms and signs may not be accompanied by a rise in intra-cerebral pressure. (Hakansson 1966.)

Pyrexia

This has been observed in a number of patients. The mechanism remains unclear.

Alopecia

This occurs in all the patients receiving whole brain radiation but the doses given usually allow regrowth of hair provided the patient live long enough.

LENGTH OF TIME TAKEN RELATIVE TO SURVIVAL TIME

In patients who survive only for a short period long treatment time is a significant side effect which must be taken into account when planning treatment.

CONTRA-INDICATIONS TO TREATMENT BY RADIATION ALONE

A number of series reporting surgical treatment for cerebral metastases have shown that there is an appreciable number of patients operated on for apparent metastases who have turned out to have other, ofter benign conditions for which whole brain radiation would be quite inappropriate (Raskind et al 1971, Haar and Patterson 1972). For this reason, radiation is contra-indicated if there is any doubt about the nature of the intra-cerebral lesion.

The same surgical series have reported a very small number of cures when excision has been performed for a solitary cerebral metastasis which has arisen some time after the cure of the primary tumour. Patients coming into this category may, therefore, be considered for craniotomy. Patients in neurological Class 4 who fail to respond to high dose Dexamethasone therapy have been shown to respond very poorly and for short periods only to cerebral radiation and it is doubtful whether it is worth treating the majority of these cases.

RESULTS OF TREATMENT

Survival

Median survival in the majority of reported series is in the order of 5-6 months and ranges from 3-9 months. At one year, 10-15% of patients are still alive and several series report approximately 5% of patients surviving for more than two years.

Quality of Survival

For patients with distressing neurological disability mere prolongation of life is of little value and quality of survival must be judged by the length of time for which symptoms remain controlled. This has been analysed by Order et al (1968) who have shown that the longer a patient survives the more likely they are to develop a recurrence of their presenting symptoms so that while 79% of surviving patients remain improved at 3 months only 31% of those

surviving to one year remain improved. In general the
duration of remission of symptoms is 1-2 months less than
the overall survival. The cause of death in approximately
70% of these patients is uncontrolled cerebral metastases.
Many patients have evidence of metastases elsewhere except
for lung cancer cases in which 75% may die without other
clinical evidence of metastases (Hendrickson 1975).

Patients who have responded well to a first course of
palliative whole brain radiation may sometimes benefit from
a second course of treatment. Approximately 45% will have
a second response with a median survival of 4 months.

FACTORS INFLUENCING RESPONSE TO WHOLE BRAIN RADIATION

Initial Neurological Status

Patients in good neurological and physical condition at
the time of treatment do better than those in poor condition.
Median survival for Class 1 patients is 30 weeks, for Class
4 patients 5 weeks (Hendrickson 1975, Seminars of Oncology).
This does not necessarily reflect a better response to
treatment in Class 1 patients but merely identifies them as
a good prognostic group.

Histology of Primary Tumour

There is little correlation between histology and response in the majority of secondaries from lung and breast
cancer although there is a suggestion that breast cancer
cases do a little better. For the less common tumours
sensitive secondaries such as those from Chorion carcinoma
may be expected to respond to treatment much better than
resistant tumours such as melanoma and renal cancer which
generally respond rather poorly.

RADIATION DOSE/TIME FACTORS

There is little evidence from the literature that higher
doses result in improved survival. Assessment is made
difficult however, by the fact that most studies report a
heterogenous collection of patients and that survival is

92

not solely determined by the outcome of cerebral radiation.

CONCLUSION

If all patients with cerebral metastases are accepted
for palliative whole brain radiotherapy approximately 20%
will fail to complete the prescribed course of treatment but
of the remainder 80% will get complete or partial relief of
symptoms. For many, control of symptoms is however, likely
to be short lived with the duration of remission 3-4 months
before return of the presenting symptoms. A few patients
may however, live for 2 years or more with a good quality of
life and the opportunity of achieving good long term palliation like this should not be missed. It is difficult to
predict which patients are likely to benefit most treatment
but it seems that fit patients in neurological Class 1 are
likely to do well and that complete relief of headaches and
convulsions will occur in approximately 60% of patients.
At the other extreme patients in neurological Class 4 and
those with radio-resistant tumours generally do badly and
there is little to be gained by treating all such cases.

REFERENCES
1. Haar, F. and Patterson, R.H., Surgery for metastatic
   intra-cranial neoplasm. Cancer 30:1241-1245, 1972
2. Hakansson, C.H., Effect of irradiation of brain tumours
   on ventricular fluid pressure. Acta Radiol (Ther) 6:22-
   32, 1967
3. Harwood, A.R., Simpson, W.J., Radiation therapy of cerebral metastases: A randomized prospective clinical trial.
   Int J Rad Oncol Biol Phys 2:1091-1094, 1977
4. Hendrickson, F.R., Radiation therapy of metastatic
   tumours. Semin Oncol 2,1:43-46, 1975
5. Hindo, W.A., De Trana, F.A., Lee, M.S., Hendrickson,
   F.R., Large dose increment radiation in treatment of
   cerebral metastases. Cancer 26:138-141, 1970
6. Kramer, S., Hendrickson, F.R., Zelen, M., Schotz, W.,
   Therapeutic trials in the management of metastatic
   brain tumours by different time/dose fraction schemes

of radiation therapy. Natl Cancer Inst Monogr 46:213-221, 1979

7. Order, S.E., Hellmann, S., Von Essen, C.F., Kligerman, M.M., Improvement in quality of survival following whole brain irradiation for brain metastasis. Radiology 91:149-153, 1969

8. Raskind, R., Weiss, S.R., Manning, J.J., Wermuth, R.E., Survival after surgical excision of single metastatic brain tumours. Radiology 111:2, 323-328, 1971

9. Young, D.F., Posner, J.B., Chu, F., Nisce, L., Rapid course radiation therapy of cerebral metastases: Results and complications. Cancer 34:1069-1076, 1974

8. RADIOTHERAPY IN EPIDURAL SPINAL CORD COMPRESSION

W.M.H. van Woerkom-Eykenboom

SUMMARY

There are different opinions on the treatment of cord
compression by epidural metastases. If there are only
early symptoms and signs, irradiation gives the best
results. High doses of dexamethasone are indicated. It
will be shown that irradiation and high doses of dexamethasone can give "unexpectedly" good or bad results.
The differences in opinion on treatment of cord compression by epidural metastases deserve to remain.

When the diagnosis epidural spinal cord compression due
to metastatic disease is established, it is often questionable as to which treatment will benefit the patient
most. Frequently the desired result is not obtained and
often the outcome is different to that which was expected. On the one hand it is known that if there are
serious neurological signs such as paraplegia, major
sensory loss or bladder disfunction the probability of
a successful response to treatment is very small. On the
other hand patients who are ambulatory at the onset of
treatment, have the best outcome. This is why early
diagnosis and prompt treatment are important. Both neurosurgeons and radiotherapists claim the best results when
utilizing these criteria.

However, it is evident that for a number of patients
treatment does not lead to improvement. This is reflec-
ted by the frequently occuring differences of opinions
on how to treat epidural spinal cord compression due to
metastatic disease. The criteria which we use to deter-
mine whether a patient will benefit from radiation therapy

are shown in table I.

Radiotherapy is always given together with high dosis of dexamethasone with the aim of preventing further clinical deterioration. The sense of well being which the patient feels (due to the dexamethasone) does not mean that there is an accompanying improvement in the neurological status.

TABLE I

Radiotherapy is given when the patient presents with:
1. known primary tumor
2. established metastatic disease
3. radiosensitive tumor
4. slow progression or minimal signs
5. incomplete block on myelogram
6. laminectomy

It is doubtful whether radiotherapy is the first choice of treatment when there is:
1. a not radiosensitive tumor
2. rapid progression or major signs
3. complete block on myelogram

There is no indication to use radiotherapy when:
1. maximum radiation dose is given followed by relapse
2. general sick patient with short life expectancy

Radiotherapy is discontinued if there are signs of progress of the disease process 48 - 72 hours after the onset of radiotherapy (emergency laminectomy is indicated).

The dose of radiotherapy we give varies from 3000 rad/2 weeks to 4500 rad/3 - $3\frac{1}{2}$ weeks depending on the nature of the tumor and eventually the response of the primary tumor to radiotherapy. To illustrate these indications I would like to show you the procedures which were followed in four patients.

Case 1 A 32 year old female was treated for Hodgkin
disease stage II A with total nodal irradiation
and had no active Hodgkin disease during four
years. She developped radicular pain, sensory
loss and bladder disfunction (within $\pm$ 1 week) but
was ambulatory at the time of treatment. The X-ray
of the thoracic spine was negative. On the myelogram there was a complete extradural block at the
level of T7. Treatment consisted of dexamethasone
and radiotherapy. After receiving a radiation dose
of 600 rad clinical deterioration occurred and the
patient was referred to the neurosurgeon for laminectomy. She became paraplegic; histology showed
malignant schwannoma. She died of lungmetastases
due to malignant schwannoma eight months later.
It is in retrospect questionable as to whether
this treatment was correct. We were under the impression that we had to deal with established metastatic disease. It became clear that it was not
established metastatic disease and the tumor was
not a radiosensitive one. The conclusion is that
a false diagnosis was made and the question arises
as to how this can be avoided. Your suggestions
are welcome.

Case 2 A 33 year old male was treated for Hodgkin disease
stage IV A with chemotherapy (MOPP). At the time
of spinal cord compression he had active Hodgkin
disease. He had pain, sensory loss, bladder disfunction and motor weakness, but was able to walk.
The X-ray of the thoracic spine showed a sclerotic
T9. On the myelogram a complete, extradural block
was present at the level of T9. Treatment consisted
of high dosage of dexamethasone combined with
radiotherapy. After several treatments had been
given clinical deterioration occurred and laminectomy was performed. Histology showed Hodgkin
disease, highly fibrotic tissue.

He died of Hodgkin disease ten months later.
Was this treatment correct? Was this a radiotherapy resistent Hodgkin disease? We thought rightly
of Hodgkin disease, which is a radiosensitive
tumor, but we were probably dealing with a radiotherapy resistent Hodgkin disease possibly due to
previously given chemotherapy.

Case 3 A 22 year old male treated for Hodgkin disease
stage III B with chemotherapy developped spinal
cord compression during a period in which he had
recurrent Hodgkin disease. He had gait ataxia.
The X-ray of the thoracic spine was negative. A
complete extradural block was found at level
T3 - T4. The treatment consisted of dexamethasone
and radiotherapy. Clinical deterioration occurred
within two days. The patient was referred to the
neurosurgeon. He became paraplegic. Histology
showed malignant schwannoma. He died of lungmetastases due to malignant schwannoma six months
later. Was this treatment correct? In view of the
missed diagnosis it was not correct. We thought
we were dealing with active Hodgkin disease, which
is a radiosensitive tumor. It became evident that
we were not dealing with established metastatic
disease and further the tumor was radio-insensi-
tive. Who could have made the right diagnosis and
who should have given the correct treatment?

Case 4 A 51 year old male - in whom the diagnosis lungcarcinoma was made - had been treated with chemotherapy because of pleuritis carcinomatosa. He developped backpain with radicular pain and sensory
loss. He was able to walk. X-ray of the thoracic
spine showed metastases with destruction in T4, T5
and T6. A complete extradural block was shown on
the myelogram. Treatment consisted of dexamethasone
and radiotherapy. During treatment the symptoms and

neurological signs disappeared. He remained ambulatory and at present is alive and still on chemotherapy. Was this treatment correct? In any case a
good result. We were confronted with metastases of
lungcarcinoma, a less radiosensitive tumor and a
complete block on the myelogram.

In patients with systemic cancer suspicion of epidural
spinal cord compression must always be present. Early
diagnosis in patients with minimal symptoms of neurological signs and prompt treatment give the optimal chance for
good results. Backpain is an important symptom to which we
pay too little attention. Radiotherapy is useful in the
treatment of neoplastic epidural spinal cord compression.
It is to be hoped that in the near future a uniform and
better schedule and new ways for treatment of neoplastic
epidural spinal cord compression will be implemented.
     We may imagine that we know how to treat patients
with neoplastic epidural spinal cord compression but in
my opinion patients, when confronted with the poor results
of our treatment may well have other ideas.

REFERENCES

1. Apuzzo, M.L.J.; Weiss, M.H.; Minassian, H.V.:
   Epidural spinal metastases;
   factors related to selection of cases for decompressive
   laminectomy
   Bull. Los Angeles neurol. Soc. 42: 63/70, 1978

2. Bruckman, J.E.; Bloomer, W.D.:
   Management of spinal cord compression
   Semin. Oncol. 5, 135/140, 1978

3. Crue, B.L.; Felsöőry, A.:
   Discussion of the indication for decpmpressive laminec-
   tomy in epidural spinal metastasis.
   Bull. Los Angeles neurol. Soc. 42, 71/76, 1978

4. Gilbert, H.; Apuzzo, M.L.J.; Marshal, L.; Kagan, A.R.;
   Crue, B.L.; Wagner, J.; Fuchs, K.; Rush, J.; Rao, A.;
   Nussbaum, H.; Chan, P.:
   Neoplastic epidural spinal cord compression;
   a current perspective
   JAMA 240: 2771/2773, 1978

5. Gilbert, R.W.; Kim, J.H.; Posner, J.B.:
   Epidural spinal cord compression from metastatic tumor;
   diagnosis and treatment
   Ann. Neurol. 3, 40/51, 1978

6. Hildebrand, J.
   Lesions of the nervous system in cancer patients
   New York, Raven 1978
   E.O.R.T.C. Monograph Serie, Vol. 5

7. Marshall, L.F.; Langfitt, T.W.:
   Combined therapy for metastatic extradural tumors of
   the spine
   Cancer 40, 2067/2077, 1977

8. Meyer, E.:
   Compressio medullae ten gevolge van wervelmetastasen;
   over de vraag naar het nut van decomprimerende lami-
   nectomieën
   Dissertatie Nijmegen, 1977

9. Posner, J.B.:
   Management of central nervouw system metastases
   Semin. Oncol. 4, 81/91, 1977

10. Posner, J.B.
    Spinal cord metastasis/ compression
    Course in Neuro-Oncology. -Memorial Sloan-Kettering
    Centre,
    New York, 1977

9. EPIDURAL SPINAL CORD COMPRESSION FROM METASTATIC TUMOR: AN ANALYSIS OF EIGHTY-THREE PATIENTS TREATED WITH RADIATION THERAPY AND STEROIDS

H.S. Greenberg

At Memorial Sloan-Kettering Cancer Center epidural cord compression is the second most frequent neurologic metastatic complication of cancer, only cerebral metastases occurring more frequently.

The treatment of epidural spinal cord compression due to metastatic cancer is unsatisfactory. In the best reported series, less than 2/3 of the patients maintain or regain ambulation, and in most series the ambulation rate after treatment is 50% or less. When large series are reported, the results are similar whether the patient has undergone decompressive laminectomy followed by radiation therapy or has been treated with radiation therapy alone. Work with an experimental tumor model of epidural spinal cord compression in the rat suggested that high doses of dexamethasone accompanied by radiation therapy delivered in dose fractionations that are somewhat higher than those conventionally used might be more efficacious than our previous protocol. Therefore, we undertook a prospective study of patients with epidural spinal cord compression from metastatic tumor using high dose dexamethasone and a new radiation fractionation course.

In this study, spinal cord or cauda equina compression was considered to be present if there was a complete or greater than 80% obstruction of the subarachnoid space at lumbar myelography. If a complete block was present cisternal or lateral C2 puncture was performed to define the upper level of the block. In the 21-month period from October 1976 to July 1978 137 patients with spinal cord or cauda equina compression were treated at Memorial Sloan-Kettering Cancer

Center. Ten patients underwent decompressive lamanectomy, 5 of these were previously irradiated to tolerance for spinal cord compression, in 3 no primary diagnosis has been made and tissue was needed. One with pancreatic carcinoma was operated on because his physicians believed that the tumor would be resistant to radiation therapy, and the tenth patient was operated on because of worsening clinical symptoms during the course of radiation therapy. Forty-four patients were excluded from the study either because they had received prior radiation therapy to the sight of their lesion or their radio-therapists selected a fractionation schedule different from the protocol. Eighty-three patients were treated according to the new protocol which is seen in Table 1.

When the clinical or radiologic diagnosis of epidural cord compression were made, either before or immediately after myelography, an intravenous bolus of 100 mg of dexamethasone was injected. The patient was then continued on a dose of 96 mg of dexamethasone in four divided doses for two days, and then tapered according to the schedule seen in Table 1.

TABLE 1.   **treatment of spinal cord compression**

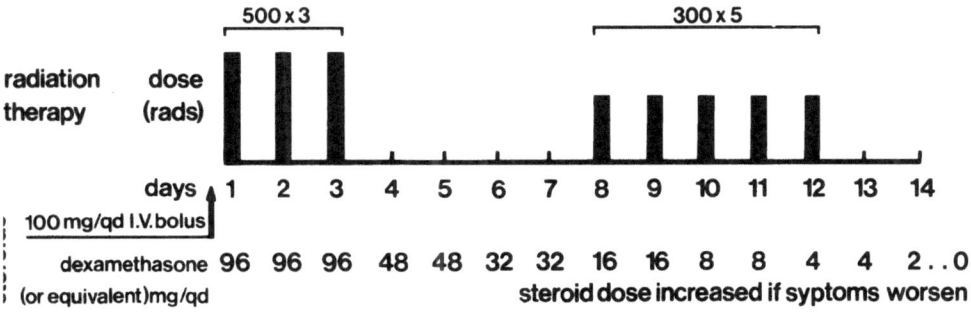

This consisted of a halving of the dose every two days with discontinuation of therapy two days following completion of radiation therapy. If the patient's clinical condition worsened at anytime during the tapering of the dose, the dose was raised to the next higher one and maintained for 48 hours before the tapering schedule was resumed again. Radiation therapy was begun within two hours of myelography at a dose of 500 rads to a posterior port centered on the site of the block and encompassing two vertebral bodies above and below the block. The 500 rads dose was given daily for three consecutive days, followed by a four-day rest and then 300 rads given daily over five consecutive days. Refluorcopy myelography was usually performed at the end of treatment and again two months following treatment.

Patients were divided into four grades, based on motor function when first examined by the neurologist. Grade 1 patients were ambulatory without assistance, although they might have considerable weakness of their lower extremities. There were 38 patients or 45% of the total in this category. Grade 2 patients, 24 in number, were not ambulatory but were able to move their legs against gravity in bed. Grade 3 patients, 13, were non-ambulatory and their movements were limited to flickering motions with one or groups of muscles in the lower extremities. Grade 4 patients, 8 in number, were entirely unable to move.

There were 40 males and 43 females in the series, with a mean age of 56 years. The interval between the diagnosis of cancer and development of spinal cord compression varied from one week to 23 years. Carcinoma of the breast was the most frequent primary neoplasm followed by prostatic and lung carcinomas. In the present series only 3 patients had a lymphoproliferative disorder which is a marked decrease from previous series. This may be due to the fact that patients with lymphoma frequently received mantle radiation for their lymphoma. This may prevent the development of spinal cord compression and also precludes the use of our protocol because these areas of the neuraxis have frequently been previously irradiated.

The cervical spinal cord was the site of compression in 12 patients or 15%, the thoracic cord in 59 or 70% and lumbar cord or cauda equina in 12 - 15%. Because our previous studies did not show that the outcome of cauda equina compression was different from epidural cord compression, the two entities are considered together.

The clinical symptoms of spinal cord compression were present from one-half day to two years prior to diagnosis and pain was the presenting symptom in 92% of cases, preceding other symptoms by a medium time of four weeks. In five patients (6%) weakness of the lower extremities was the presenting sign and in one patient each, ataxia or sensory loss was the initial complaint. At the time of diagnosis fifty-eight patients or 70% complained of weakness and approximately 50% of the patients complained of sensory loss or autonomic dysfunction. In 9 patients, all with thoracic lesions, four with a complete block, pain was the only symptom or sign when they presented with a block. At the time of diagnosis 72 patients or 91%, had radiographically documented metastases to the vertebral body at the level of compression.

The results of treatment with respect to pain relief were that thirty-nine of 61 patients (63%) questioned about pain relief had dramatic reduction of pain the first day following therapy. Six patients had complete relief of pain after the 100 mg intravenous dose of dexamethasone, before the first dose of radiation therapy was administered. Such dramatic relief of pain was entirely different from our experience using conventional doses of steroids or radiation therapy without steroids. This relief of pain was documented by a substantial reduction of narcotic requirements on the first day following steroid treatment. A few patients became tremulous and showed signs of narcotic withdrawal after voluntary and abrupt discontinuation of their pain medication. Pain relief was also achieved in 13 of the remaining 22 patients by the end of radiation therapy yielding an overall 82% pain relief. Unfortunately there was no correlation between immediate pain relief and successful treatment to outcome. Twenty-three of thirty-nine patients

or 59% with immediate pain relief eventually became ambulatory, which is similar to the series as a whole where 57% of
patients were ambulatory following treatment. Of the grade
1 patients, those ambulatory at outset, 34 out of 38 or 89%,
remained ambulatory. Of the 24 grade 2 patients who were
not ambulatory but had antigravity function, 10 out of 24 or
42% regained ambulation. In those with only a flicker of
movement or grade 3, 3 out of 13 patients regained ambulation
None of the 8 patients who were paraplegic regained ambulation.

No patient with lung carcinoma improved from a non-ambulatory to an ambulatory status with treatment. Four patients,
two with lung and two with prostatic deteriorated from ambulatory at the onset of treatment to grade 2 or 3 with treatment.

Next considering the treatment response by tumor type 52%
of breast cancer patients were ambulatory at the completion
of treatment. Surprisingly, patients with prostatic and
renal tumors, generally not considered highly radiosensitive
had a 67% rate of ambulation. Patients with lung carcinoma
did poorly with only 27% ambulatory at the completion of
treatment. The data with lung carcinoma are consistent with
those previously recorded in the literature. When the tumors
are divided into two groups, those considered to be highly
sensitive to radiation therapy such as lymphoma, myeloma, or
neuroblastoma, and those considered to be less sensitive,
the ambulation rate was 62% for the sensitive tumors and 55%
for the less radiosensitive tumors.

Sphincter involvement with urinary incontinence or
constipation was associated with a poor prognosis. Thirty-
seven of 83 patients or 45% had sphincter involvement, and
of these only 27% regained ambulation. Return of sphincter
function paralleled and often preceded the return of motor
function. In patients grade 2 or 3 after treatment,
sphincter function often returned during their radiation
therapy, enabling the foley catheter to be removed. In
patients who were paraplegic or grade 4, sphincter control
did not return.

Serious complications of corticosteroids occurred in only one patient, who, on the fourth day following treatment developed an acute abdomen from a ruptured duodenal ulcer. He recovered following laparotomy. No other patient suffered serious complications. Some patients complained of insomnia and tremulousness and several became euphoric.

Two elements in this protocol for the treatment of spinal cord compres.-sion differ from those used previously. The first is the dose of dexamethasone delivered by bolus and alsoorally over the first several days, and the second is the radiation fractionation course. Both of these were chos chosen on the basis of animal studies of Ushio et al from our laboratory, which suggested that high dose dexamethasone improved neurologic function beginning the first day after treatment and maintained improvement for 3 to 4 days, even when the animals were not irradiated. Dexamethasone, however, did not maintain improvement permanently, the animals all relapsed unless radiation therapy was delivered. The second element of that study indicated that improvement in ambulation was initially directly proportional to the dose of radiation therapy given. Thus, 100 rads in a single dose improved ambulation in animals to a greater degree than did 500 rads given in three doses or 200 rads given over 8 doses. However, maintenance of improvement was superior when the animals were given 500 rads in three doses rather than one of the other two fractionation protocols. For that reason we selected a protocol where a high dose of radiation therapy was delivered fairly rapidly over three days and a consolidation course was given over five days after a four-day rest period. The radiobiologic rationale is that high doses are more efficient in inducing rapid tumor cell cytolysis and improving reoxygenation because of tumor shrinkage. Reoxygenation theoretically helps eliminate the hypoxic fraction of solid tumors, making the tumor more susceptible to the RT which follows the rest period.

The results of steroid treatment were encouraging. With minimal morbidity most patients had rapid and complete amelioration of pain, thus allowing them to be considerably more comfortable during the days while they were being treated with radiation therapy. The side effects of steroid therapy were mild and probably not of greater frequency than with patients treated with more conventional doses of steroids Thus, the use of high dose steroids at the time the diagnosis is first established seems warranted, at least for the relief of pain. The effects of steroids on motor function were difficult to assess because all patients were radiated almost immediately following myelography, and one cannot draw any conclusions about them from this study. Results from the alteration of the radiation therapy protocol were disappointing. 57% of patients were ambulatory at the completion of treatment which is a slight but not significant increase in ambulation rate after treatment, compared to the study of Gilbert et al where 45% of patients were ambulatory.

10. GROWTH RETARDATION AS A COMPLICATION OF RADIOTHERAPY IN CHILDREN WITH BRAIN TUMOURS

R.P. Droog, H. Behrendt, P.A. Voûte

Since the use of radiotherapy in the treatment of
children with braintumours the prognosis of these patients
has significantly improved. On the whole it concerns
children with medulloblastoma, astrocytoma and ependymoma.
A long-term recurrent free survival period is reached
nowadays with 30 - 50% of these patients. Some of these
children survive with moderate to serious neurological
damage, while others are cured without any obvious sign of
damage from the tumour or the treatment. As the follow up
period of these children becomes longer and more children
survive, approximately half of these long-term survivors
appear to have the phenomenon of growth retardation. The
growth curve of these children dips immediately after
surgical and radiotherapeutical treatment. An example of
this growth disturbance is shown in figure 1.
Endocrinological investigation of these patients shows a
lack of Growth Hormone while in most cases the other
pituitary hormones are normally present. There are reasons
to assume that not the tumour itself, but the radiotherapy
is the cause of the development of the growth hormone
deficiency. There are several reasons to substantiate that:
First   - If the tumour itself gave rise to diminished
            growth hormone production, the growth in a
            number of patients would already be disturbed

108

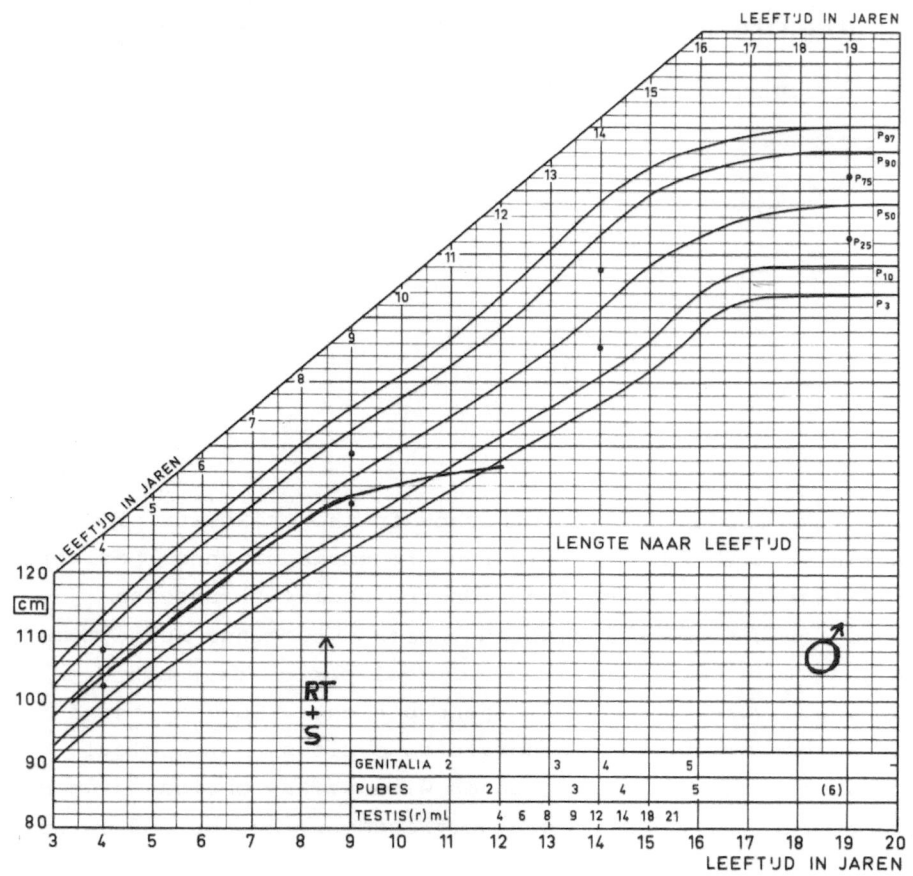

Figure 1: The growth diagram shows the
normal distribution of the Dutch population
as regards length. On the horizontal axis
the age is set and on the vertical axis the
length. The growth curve of an 8½ year old
boy is shown. He was treated with surgery (S)
and radiotherapy (R) and showed shortly after
that a drop of his growth curve.

before the start of the therapy. However, the growth disorder always occurs after the treatment, also in children with braintumours which grow slowly.

Secondly - It has been shown that the existence or non-existence of growth hormone deficiency correlates to the irradiation dose used. Children with braintumours receive a radiation dose of 5000 rad on the skull and growth disorders are frequent in these patients. On the other hand no growth disorders are seen in children with acute leukaemia who receive for prophylactic reasons irradiation on the whole skull with a radiation dose of 2500 rad given in 2½ weeks. If the irradiation dose is more than 2500 rad growth disorders can be expected.

The third argument for the growth retarding effect of radiotherapy is shown in figure 2.

We must realize that this situation, in which growth hormone deficiency arises as a consequence of the therapy, is completely different from that seen in children with craniopharyngioma, in which pituitary insufficiency arises as a consequence of tumour invasion into the pituitary. In these cases we mostly find a deficiency of several pituitary hormones.

For the treatment of children with a growth disorder based on a growth hormone deficiency, substitution with Human Growth Hormone is indicated. An example of the result of substitution therapy is given in figure 3 which shows the growth curve of the patient of figure 1 after starting growth hormone substitution.

Conclusions

1. Growth disorders are found in half of the children treated for a brain tumour with radiotherapy.
2. In these children a growth hormone deficiency is found in most cases.

110

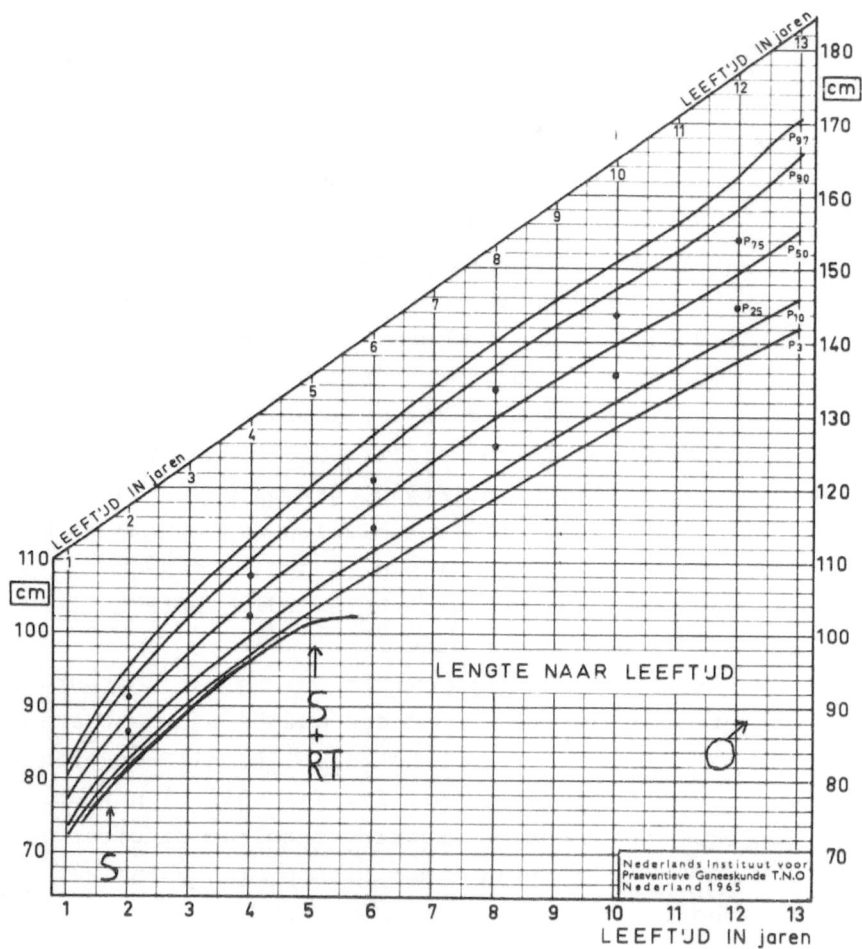

Figure 2: S = surgery, R = radiotherapy.
This growth curve belongs to a boy who was
operated for a braintumour at 1½ year of age.
Macroscopically the whole tumour was removed.
Because of his age no radiotherapy was given.
At the age of 5 he had a relapse of his tumour.
He was then operated and given radiotherapy.
After that he developed a drop of his growth
curve.

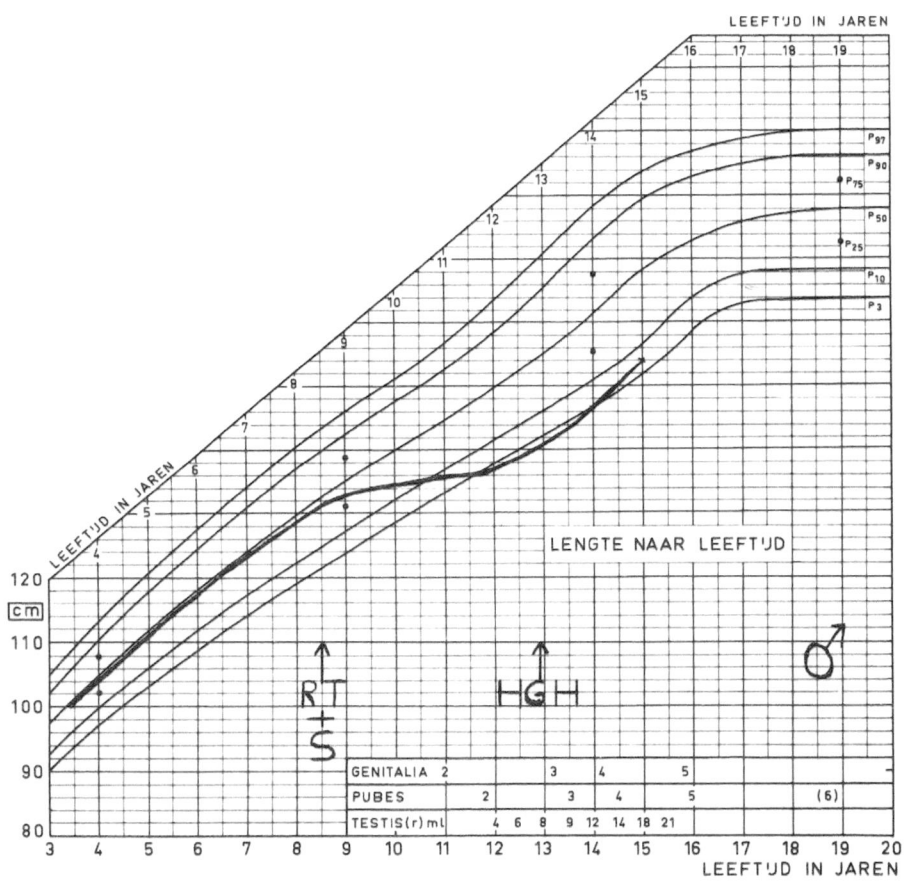

Figure 3: H.G.H. = Human Growth Hormone,
S = surgery, R = radiotherapy. Growth
curve of the patient of figure 1 after
starting substitution therapy.

3. The growth hormone deficiency is probably caused by the radiotherapy and not by the tumour itself.
4. Growth retardation is not found if the radiation dose is less than 2500 rad.

The foregoing illustrates clearly the need to treat children with malignant diseases in or in close cooperation with a centre for paediatric oncology.

REFERENCES

1. Czernichow P., O. Cachin, R. Rappaport, F. Flamant D. Sarrazin and O. Schweisguth, Sequelles endocriniennes des irradiations de la tête et du cou pour tumeurs extracraniennes. Arch Franc Péd 34, CLIV - CLXIV 1977
2. Perry-Keene D.A., J.F. Connelly, R.A. Young, H.N.B. Wettenhall and F.I.R. Martin, Hypothalamic hypo-pituitarism following external radiotherapy for tumours distant from the adenohypophysis. Clinical endocrinology 5, 373-380, 1976
3. Samaan N.A., M.M. Bakdash, J.B. Caderao et al, Hypo-pituitarism after external irradiation. Annals of Internal Medicine 83, 771-777, 1975
4. Shalet S.M., C.G. Beardwell, P.H. Morris Jones and D. Pearson, Growth hormone deficiency after treatment of acute leukaemia in children. Arch of Dis in Childhood 51, 489-493, 1976
5. Shalet S.M., C.G. Beardwell, D. Pearson and P.H. Morris Jones, The effect of varying doses of cerebral irradiation on growth hormone production in childhood. Clin. Endocrinology 5, 287-290, 1976
6. Shalet S.M., C.G. Beardwell, J.A. Twomey, P.H. Morris Jones and D. Pearson, Endocrine function following the treatment of acute leukaemia in childhood. Journal of Paediatrics vol 90, 6, 920-923, June 1977
7. Shalet S.M., C.G. Beardwell, B.M. Aarons, D. Pearson and P.H. Morris Jones, Growth impairment in children treated for brain tumours. Arch of Dis in Childhood 53, 491-494, 1978
8. Shalet S.M., D.A. Price, C.G. Beardwell et al, Normal growth despite abnormality of growth hormone secretion in children treated for acute leucaemia. Journal of Paediatrics vol 94, 5, 719-722, 1979
9. Sunderman C.R., H.A. Pearson, Growth effects of long-term anti-leukaemic therapy. Journal of Paediatrics vol 75, 6, 1058-1062.
10. Swift P.G.F., P.J. Kearney, R.G. Dalton et al, Growth and hormonal status of children treated for acute lymfoblastic leucaemia. Arch of Dis in Childhood 53, 890-894, 1978

11. NEUROSURGICAL MANAGEMENT OF SPINAL METASTASES CAUSING CORD AND CAUDA EQUINA COMPRESSION

E. Meyer

SUMMARY

In the treatment of certain tumor types, neurosurgical management (laminectomy) is bound to fail. In the handling of other tumor types, expectations should focus on hormonal, radiological and cytostatic treatment; in these cases laminectomy might be of supportive value. It is of importance to bear in mind that, in the presence of severe kyphosis, laminectomy has little or no effect because the cord is taut over the gibbus and therefore cannot be decompressed by laminectomy. Another fact to be borne in mind is that laminectomy can unfavourably influence the stability of the vertebral column.

The results obtained in a study from a hundred patients are very disappointing at least as far as the restoration of neurological dysfunctions is concerned. Early diagnosis is the key factor in improving results in neoplastic epidural spinal cord compression.

The vertebral column, it has been established, is a particularly favourable site for metastases of a malignant process. It is believed that metastases are demonstrable in several vertebrae in two-thirds of the cases of spinal metastases. Most lesions are found in the thoracic segment of the spine. Ossophilic tumors mainly arise from malignant processes in the breast, prostate, thyroid, kidney and lung. In 50% of the cases the metastasis is the first symptom of a malignant process.

Table 1.

	male	female	mean age in years
Lung carcinoma	19	-	55,6
Breast carcinoma	1	19	54,5
Testis carcinoma	6	-	34,8
Gastrointestinal carcinoma	3	5	60,7
Hypernephroma	6	3	53,1
Thyroid carcinoma	2	4	53,8
Bladder carcinoma	1	-	68
Palatum carcinoma	1	1	46
Uterus and adnexa carcinoma	-	3	52
Melanosarcoma	-	2	51
Prostatic carcinoma	13	-	66,3
Rhabdomyosarcoma	1	-	32
Unknown	2	8	55,2
	55	45	

Pressure exerted on the cord or on radicular arteries by tumor growth outside the vertebral body or vertebral arch, or by a pathological fracture, gives rise to changes in the general circulatory, humoral and cellular processes. These processes cause the functional disorders which manifest themselves as paraplegia. Due to the vulnerability of the spinal cord, these processes quickly become irreversible so that decompression can no longer be effective.

Much has been written about spinal metastases, and about their surgical therapy. However, the results of all these studies, and particularly the follow-up results, vary widely and are evidently dependent on the personality of the investigator.

Moreover, the incidence of cord compression as a result of spinal metastases is not sufficiently high to obtain reliable statistics. Törma (1957) reported on a large series of 250 patients from five hospitals over a period of 30 years, but he lumped together all tumor types, benign and malignant, primary and secundary, systemic diseases, etc.

Some specialists, internists and/or neurologists, often have only one wish once they have diagnosed the neurological complications of spinal metastases: to transfer the patient to a surgical
department, because they do not know what to do with a paraplegic.

Some surgeons regard even the slightest postoperative improvement
as a success, and quickly have the patient transferred to a nursing home .... out of their sight.

Table 2. Results of laminectomy (literature reports)

				Improvement
Alexander	1956	22 pat.		27.2%
Smith	1965	49 "		33.0%
Vieth	1965	34 "		38.2%
Rogers	1969	60 "		43.0%
			long term	20.0%
Raichle	1970	22 "		32.0%
White	1971	226 "		36.0%
Store	1973	23 "		30.0%
Meijer	1977	86 "		15.0%
Gorter	1978	31 "		38.7%
Livingston	1978	100 "		58.0%
			long term	40.0%

A casuistic analysis reveals that surgical therapy has little or
no effect, and that some patients are worse off after an operation than before. It is therefore highly questionable whether the
results warrant routine performance of laminectomy.

It is obvious that many of the data presented in the literature
must be taken with a grain of salt.

The most readily understandable tables are those which divide the
patients into a preoperative and a postoperative group, and into
walking and bed-ridden patients. A study of these tables disclos-
es that a laminectomy can be dangerous, and in fact can cause aggravation of the neurological symptoms!

Table 3 (Wright 1963)

Preoperative status		Postoperative status		
		paraplegic	paretic	ambulant
paraplegic	18	16	2	0
paretic	49	16	15	18
ambulant	10	2	7	10

Table 4 (White c.s. 1971)

Preoperative status		Postoperative status	
ambulant	42	ambulant	64%
		not ambulant	22%
		paraplegic	14%
paretic (not ambulant)	155	ambulant	34%
		not ambulant	47%
		paraplegic	19%
paraplegic	29	ambulant	10%
		not ambulant	14%
		paraplegic	76%

In our series, too, a fair number of complications developed:

    2 patients died during or short after the operation (2%)
    7 patients showed more neurological symptoms (7%)
    10 patients had a trombosis or embolia (10%)
    2 patients had a postoperative psychoses (2%)
    3 patients had a woundinfection (3%)
    1 patient had an entmetastasis in the skin (1%)

The fact of the matter simply is that little can be done about a
spinal metastasis because in most cases several vertebrae are affected, and metastases are likely to be present elsewhere in the
organism as well. Besides general therapeutic measures, every

possible effort has to be made to prevent the possible consequence of paraplegia. We all know how terribly paraplegics must suffer, with decubitus, bladder and rectum problems, etc.. Completely dependent on other people. And this in the terminal phase of
their life.

I agree with **Marshall and Langfitt** (1977), who advised the following therapeutic measures in the case of a spinal metastasis which
causes pain or even the slightest signs of cord compression:
1. large doses of corticosteroids; that is to say, for example,
   40 mg dexamethasone per day (this medication is believed to
   reduce angiogenic oedema and may also have an oncolytic effect)
2. radiotherapy and chemotherapy
3. adrenalectomy and hypophysectomy can exert a very favourable
   influence on hormone-dependent processes, and the same applies
   to ovariectomy. The pain, too, can thus be alleviated. Carcinoma of the prostate sometimes shows a favourable response to
   castration and administration of oestrogens.
When these measures prove to be insufficient, an operation should
be performed immediately, before total cord dysfunction develops.
It is to be born in mind, however, that chemotherapy may give
rise to haematological changes which preclude surgical therapy.
The guidelines I mentioned are acceptable, and only an anterior
approach to the affected vertebra is in principle an even better
therapy. The anterior approach, after all, ensures radical resection of the evil and also abolishes the ventral compression of
the cord. This therapy is more logical than dorsal resection of
one or several vertebral arches (laminectomy), and should therefore be preferred if it is technically feasible. A prerequisite
is that the vertebral metastasis responsible for the neurological
complications is the only demonstrable metastasis and that the
neurological complications are not too serious and not too long-
standing. Another prerequisite for this major operation is a life
expectancy of at least a few months.
We have so far largely confined ourselves to patients with only
slight signs of cord compression. Unfortunately, patients of this

type are not often presented; we are still being confronted with
many patients who have been totally paralysed in bed for a week
or longer.

Table 5.

	Preoperative status		Postoperative status
	paraplegic	paretic	Improved:
Lung carcinoma	10	9	3
Breast carcinoma	9	11	3
Testis carcinoma	3	3	-
Gastrointestinal carcinoma	6	2	2
Hypernephroma	5	4	1
Thyroid carcinoma	2	4	1
Bladder carcinoma	-	1	-
Palatum carcinoma	-	2	2
Uterus and adnexa carcinoma	1	2	-
Melanosarcoma	1	1	-
Prostatic carcinoma	7	6	4
Rhabdomyosarcoma	-	1	1
Unknown	2	8	-
	46	54	17

17% of the patients with a compression of the medulla spinalis or
the cauda equina by a metastasis of a malignant process in a vertebra came in a better condition after a laminectomy.
But: From the paraplegic patients (46) only 4 improved (8.7%)
    From the paretic patients (54) 13 improved (24%).

The following may serve to demonstrate some of our results:
only 3 of the 19 patients with a pulmonary carcinoma metastasis
showed improvement. It is of interest that the compression in
these cases was at the lumbar area, that is to say at the level
of the cauda equina, where the results are slightly more favourable.

Only 3 of the 20 patients with a breast carcinoma metastasis showed improvement.

Four of the 13 patients with a prostatic carcinoma came in a better situation (but they also got hormonal therapy!)

Of the six patients with a testicular carcinoma metastasis, none
recovered.

In fact the results seem rather gloomy.

With some investigators I discussed the gloomy conclusions based
on their follow-up studies. When I asked them what they intended
to do with their next patients, they said: "Operate, of course,
because the patient should always be given every possible chance".

Others even maintain that, if only one out of 100 operations
leads to recovery, this single recovery makes these 100 operations worth while.

I do not agree with this. In my opinion we should look for other
criteria, and indications for surgical decompression should be
more strictly defined.

A splendid study by Gilbert, Kim and Possner (1978) of 130 patients shows that decompressive laminectomy gives no better results than other therapies. They compared a group of patients
treated by operation and postoperative radiotherapy, with a group
treated solely by radiotherapy; and they found absolutely no difference!

Many of our colleagues continue to operate, but an increasing
number of others are pointing out that surgical decompression is
useless. We have come to the conclusion that an intermediate solution is conceivable, because our follow-up showed that especially the time factor is of importance. Not the duration of the
paraplegic symptomatology, but the speed with which these symptoms develop.

Rapid development of cord compression leads to irreversible lesions, probably as a result of vascular disorders. A more insidi-
ously developing paralysis, however, can be reversed. You must be
aware that symptoms of cord compression caused by a meningeoma
or neurinoma, even if present for several months, can disappear
after tumor extirpation.

120

Table 6

	Acute (subacute) paraplegia.	Postoperative improvement.
Lung carcinoma	9	-
Breast carcinoma	7	-
Testis carcinoma	5	-
Gastrointestinal carcinoma	4	-
Hypernephroma	5	-
Thyroid carcinoma	3	-
Bladder carcinoma	1	-
Palatum carcinoma	1	-
Uterus and adnexa carcinoma	1	-
Melanosarcoma	1	-
Prostatic carcinoma	3	-
Rhabdomyosarcoma	-	-
Unknown	5	-
	45	-

Table 7

	Slow progressive paraplegic	Postoperative improvement:
Lung carcinoma	10	3
Breast carcinoma	13	3
Testis carcinoma	1	-
Gastrointestinal carcinoma	4	2
Hypernephroma	4	1
Thyroid carcinoma	3	1
Bladder carcinoma	-	-
Palatum carcinoma	1	2
Uterus and adnexa carcinoma	2	-
Melanosarcoma	1	-
Prostatic carcinoma	10	4
Rhabdomyosarcoma	1	1
Unknown	5	-
	55	17 (31%)

In the decision to resort to surgical therapy it is not only the
patient's general condition that plays a role, but also the condition of the vertebral column, on which CT-scanning and bone
scanning provide detailed information.

If we confine ourselves to problems of pain which shows little or
no response to medication, then the range of indications for surgical therapy widens.

Table 8

	Total	Pain relieved
Lung carcinoma	19	4
Breast carcinoma	20	4
Testis carcinoma	6	-
Gastrointestinal carcinoma	8	2
Hypernephroma	9	1
Thyroid carcinoma	6	1
Bladder carcinoma	1	1
Palatum carcinoma	2	-
Uterus and adnexa carcinoma	3	-
Melanosarcoma	2	-
Prostatic carcinoma	13	3
Rhabdomyosarcoma	1	-
Unknown	10	2
	100	18

Even in this respect, however, I would wish to make a plea for a
more conservative approach to these patients because experience
has taught us that careful guidance of these doomed patients often given better results than can be obtained with the scalpel.

Conclusions

It is of importance to take a careful history of patients with
pain in the back, because a malignant process in a vertebra may
be the cause.
In 50% of our patients the vertebral lesion was the first symptom
of a malignant process.
Once the process is localized by careful clinical and radiological examination, efforts may be made to influence the process by
corticosteroid medication, chemotherapy and/or radiotherapy.
If in spite of this signs of cord compression are observed and
the neurological dysfunction exacerbates and signs of paraplegia
develop, an immediate operation is necessary. An ample laminectomy is indicated, unless a ventral approach to the process is
feasible.
Paraplegia of more than 24 hours' standing which has developed

within a short time, say a few hours, requires no surgical therapy. In a few of these cases, a diagnostic laminectomy may be necessary when a vertebral puncture has remained unsuccessful.
Lumbar puncture, and therefore also lumbar myelography, is definitely inadvisable in view of the risk of herniation. Suboccipital myelography seems safer in these cases.

REFERENCES

1. Gilbert, RW, JH Kim, and JB Posner, Epidural spinal cord
   compression from metastatic tumor. Ann Neurol 3:40,1978

2. Gorter, K, Results of laminectomy in spinal cord compression
   due to tumours. Acta Neurochir,Wien 42:177, 1978

3. Livingston, KE and RG Perrin, The neurosurgical management
   of spinal metastases causing cord and cauda equina compression. J Neurosurg 49:839,1978

4. Marshall, LF and TW Langfitt, Combined therapy for metastatic extradural tumors of the spine. Cancer 40:2067, 1977

5. Meijer, E, Compressio medullae ten gevolge van wervelmetastasen. Diss Nijmegen, 1977

6. Posner, JB, J Howieson and E Cvitkovic, "Disappearing" spinal cord compression: oncolytic effect of glucocorticoids
   (and other chemotherapeutic agents) on epidural metastases
   Ann Neurol 2:409, 1977

7. Törma, T, Malignant tumours of the spine and the spinal extradural space. Acta Chir Scand , Suppl 225, 1957

8. White, WA, RH Patterson and RM Bergland, Role of surgery in
   the treatment of the spinal cord compression by metastatic
   neoplasm. Cancer 27:558, 1971

9. Wright, RL, Malignant tumors in the spinal extradural space.
   Ann Surg 157:223, 1963

12. CHEMOTHERAPY AND THE NERVOUS SYSTEM

J.B. Posner

The problems of systemic chemotherapy and its effects on both central
nervous system (CNS) neoplasms and the nervous system itself are
enormous. There are little data available (although that does not
prevent many of us from having strong opinions), and there are many
areas of controversy. What I would like to do in this discussion is
address very briefly 3 aspects of systemic chemotherapy and the CNS,
reviewing what some of the available data are and, in addition, what
some of the problems which face us in the future might be.

1. CHEMOTHERAPY OF MALIGNANT GLIOMAS

The first area is that of the chemotherapy of primary CNS tumors,
specifically malignant gliomas. In 1978 the Brain Tumor Study Group
in the United States published the results of a randomized study using
radiation therapy (RT) and 1,3-bis-(2-chloroethyl)-1-nitrosourea
(BCNU)(1): There were 4 groups of patients; all 4 groups were
operated on. One group received no further therapy; 2 other groups
received either RT or BCNU, and the 4th group both RT and BCNU.
Patients who received a maximum feasible surgical resection but no
further therapy had a median survival of about 4 months; virtually all
of them were dead in less than a year. Patients who received RT
5000-6000 rad after maximum feasible surgical resection lived longer,
although the vast majority of those patients were also dead within a
year and a half. Patients who received chemotherapy with BCNU after
surgery but without RT did not live as long as those patients who were
treated with RT. However, in the BCNU group there is a "tail" on the
survival curve indicating that a few patients are longer survivors.
The tail differentiates BCNU therapy from patients who received
operation but no further therapy. Finally, a combination of maximum

feasible surgical resection followed by RT and chemotherapy with BCNU yielded not only an increased survival over those patients who received no therapy after the surgery, but there were more long survivors, often out to and beyond 2 years.

The latest (as yet unpublished) data of the Brain Tumor Study Group indicate that a combination of RT and BCNU, which was the best arm from the previous study, yields a median survival of over a year as opposed to 4 months with surgery alone (from the previous study). After RT and chemotherapy, as many as 30% of patients in one arm were alive at 120 weeks or two and a half years after the study was undertaken. Thus, it seems clearly demonstrated by the Brain Tumor Study Group that RT is superior to surgical resection alone for the treatment of malignant gliomas and that when there is an addition of appropriate chemotherapy to the RT group, many patients survive beyond 2 years, often with a good "quality of life" during that period of time. I have no doubt that changes in chemotherapy in the future will produce longer survivors and better quality of life if we can identify appropriate drugs.

So much for primary malignant gliomas. Let us turn for a moment to the question of the chemotherapy of brain metastases, which represent a numerically much greater problem and which have already been discussed in this conference.

2. BRAIN METASTASES AND THE BLOOD-BRAIN BARRIER

I have no quantitative data to show you because there are little available in the literature (2). The question of whether the blood-brain barrier plays a role in the development and therapy of brain metastases is an important one, but the answer is still unknown. We have encountered at least one patient at Memorial Hospital in whom an asymptomatic brain metastasis from breast carcinoma was treated with doxorubicin (a drug which does not normally cross the blood-brain barrier) in whom, 2 months later (when she was still asymptomatic neurologically) the tumor had disappeared. Four months after that, in the setting of her systemic symptoms relapsing, the tumor reappeared; she died a few months later. This response is, in fact, what one might expect from an effective chemotherapeutic agent for a systemic cancer. After all, there does not appear to be a blood-brain barrier in this metastatic tumor, and if the systemic agent is effective, then it should be as effective in the brain as elsewhere in the body.

However, we have also treated another patient with an asymptomatic brain metastasis, this one from testicular carcinoma. There were multiple pulmonary metastases throughout both lung fields and an asymptomatic left frontal brain metastasis which was relatively small. Because it was asymptomatic, we elected not to give RT but to use systemic chemotherapy with one of our new multiple-drug protocols. The systemic chemotherapy was partially effective. The tumors in the lungs shrunk on an average of 30% each 2 months after chemotherapy was begun, but when the CT scan was repeated, not only had the original metastasis grown, but a larger metastasis in the right occipital region had appeared. The question is: Where was the metastasis while the patient was receiving chemotherapy? Was it protected by an intact blood-brain barrier? I have no answer to that, and there are no large series in the literature which bear on that question.

Therefore, we turned to an animal model to see if we could make a brain metastasis and to see what the effects of such a lesion would be on the blood-brain barrier (3). What we did was to inject Walker 256 carcinoma cells (this is a mammary carcinoma which originally arose spontaneously in the breast of the rat) into the carotid artery to see if the tumor would grow in the brain. What happened to the rat was that the tumor grew vigorously in the jaw and around the skull, and within a period of 3-4 weeks the animal had died of inanition, with a brain that was essentially clear of tumor. We next used the same model, but after 2 weeks (by which time there was some tumor apparent in the jaw), treating the animal with the chemotherapeutic agent cyclophosphamide, which is a water-soluble agent which is very effective against the Walker 256 tumor. About 50% of the animals we so treated were cured of all tumor. In the other 50%, however, the tumor in the jaw regressed, leaving only fibrous tissue. Aafter several weeks a tumor appeared in the brain. If the animals were not retreated, the tumor grew larger and within a month from the time of initial treatment essentially replaced the hemisphere. This experiment raises several questions. One of these is: If the cyclophosphamide was so effective in treating a large jaw tumor, why was it not effective in treating the small brain tumor which must have been present at the time the cyclophosphamide was given? The answer to that is unclear, but we began on that basis to investigate the problem of blood-brain barrier function in these tumors.

The first question we addressed is: What is the nature of the blood-brain barrier in metastatic tumors created by this model. With Dr. Ronald Blasberg at the National Institutes of Health we began to look at the blood-brain barrier using a chemical called alpha-amino-isobutyric acid (4). This is an artificial amino acid which does not cross the blood-brain barrier under normal circumstances but which crosses into brain at sites where the barrier does not exist and, once in the brain, is fixed in cells. It is picked up avidly by living cells and not further metabolized, so that if one gives C^{14}-labeled alpha-amino-isobutyric acid, one should be able to mark the site at which the blood-brain barrier is broken down. We found that when one gives C^{14}-labeled alpha-amino-isobutyric acid, one can identify the site of blood-brain barrier breakdown in the larger tumors, but very small metastatic brain tumors have a normal blood-brain barrier. This suggests the possibility that, even in patients with systemic disease and metastases to the brain, there is a time in the development of brain metastases when the blood-brain barrier may protect that tumor to some degree against systemic chemotherapeutic agents.

This experiment raises another question. What would happen if one were to break down the blood-brain barrier and try to get chemo-therapeutic agents across at a time when the tumor was protected by the barrier? Rapoport (5) developed a method for doing this. The method involves injecting hyperosmolar mannitol into the carotid artery of an animal. After hyperosmolar exposure, the blood-brain barrier is broken down for a period of 2-4 hours; large molecules, including trypan blue, can cross into the brain easily. The blood-brain barrier reconstitutes itself in about 4 hours, and the animal recovers fully. In experimental animals this is a safe procedure, and Dr. Neuwelt in Dallas has done this experiment in human beings and avers that it is a safe procedure (6).

One can also show the site of blood-brain barrier breakdown by the

use of horseradish peroxidase (7). Horseradish peroxidase with a
molecular weight of 40,000 does not cross a normal blood-brain
barrier, as shown in the unstained hemisphere, but if the blood-brain
barrier is broken down by hyperosmolar mannitol, this large molecule
easily gets across. Therefore, if we want to get water-soluble
chemotherapeutic agents into the brain of an animal or a patient, one
way of doing it would be to use this technique to break down the
blood-brain barrier, at least in one hemisphere. We have carried out
such a study in experimental animals, and the results (8) were quite
interesting. What they showed was that at least in the tumors we
used, there was no more methotrexate, a water-soluble chemotherapeutic
agent, in the tumor of the animals whose blood-brain barrier was open
than there was in the tumor of the animals whose blood-brain barrier
was not open. This affirms the original belief that, at least in
large metastatic tumors, there is no significant blood-brain barrier.
In addition, in the normal brain immediately surrounding the tumor (an
area of edema without tumor cells) there was no more methotrexate
after hyperosmolar mannitol than before, so that not only does one get
methotrexate in large quantities into the tumor, one also gets it
diffusing out into the surrounding brain in approximately equal
amounts. In the brain distant from the metastatic tumor, there was a
great deal more methotrexate after hyperosmolar mannitol than in
controls. The conclusion from this preliminary study is that one can
open the blood-brain barrier easily and get methotrexate in large
concentrations into the normal brain, but one does not get any more
methotrexate into the tumor or the edematous brain surrounding the
tumor than one would get without opening the blood-brain barrier if
the tumor were large enough to have broken down the barrier.

3. NERVOUS SYSTEM COMPLICATIONS OF SYSTEMIC CHEMOTHERAPY

The third aspect of chemotherapy I would like to discuss is: Is any
good likely to come from getting all this methotrexate into the normal
brain, or is it a bad thing? One answer is that the blood-brain
barrier has a purpose, and the purpose may be to keep out the drugs
oncologists are giving to human beings because many of those drugs are
toxic to the CNS. You are all aware of the entity of methotrexate-
induced leukoencephalopathy in patients with acute leukemia; this

topic is discussed at this conference by Dr. Price. Patients with acute leukemia who have received prophylactic RT to the brain and who received methotrexate either intrathecally, intravenously or at times even orally, can develop a disease of the white matter of the brain which can be seriously symptomatic. Patients with primary brain tumors who have been irradiated and who receive either intrathecal methotrexate or high-dose intravenous methotrexate may develop leukoencephalopathy (9,10). The same is true of patients with meningeal carcinomatosis who receive RT and intrathecal methotrexate; the encephalopathy likewise can also be significantly symptomatic. The question I want to address now is: What happens to patients who have no brain disease at all but receive high-dose intravenous methotrexate with citrovorum rescue for the treatment of, for example, osteogenic sarcoma? A small minority of these patients develop encephalopathy. The encephalopathy can be one of 2 kinds, as Dr. Jeffrey Allen at our institution has recently reported (10,11). One is an acute onset encephalopathy which usually occurs 7-14 days after a high dose of intravenous methotrexate. It often occurs after the 3rd or 4th high dose of intravenous methotrexate, but does not recur after additional doses. The signs and symptoms of this acute encephalopathy are sudden paralysis, either unilateral or bilateral, with or without focal or generalized seizures. The hemiparasis may fluctuate in severity and change location from side to side during the course of the acute illness, which lasts several days. After several days of acute neurologic dysfunction, the patient stabilizes and then may completely recover. If the patient is rechallenged with methotrexate for additional courses (remember, we are dealing with a malignant and an almost uniformly lethal tumor, so that we must go ahead and treat the patient), he does not again develop an acute encephalopathy. It seems to be a one-time occurrence in some patients who are treated with high-dose intravenous methotrexate (11). We have no idea what the predisposing factors are. None of our patients have died, so that we have no pathology. We have done CT scans and arteriograms on all of the patients, thinking of a vascular insult, but the CT scans and arteriograms are uniformly normal, although the electroencephalogram showed slow wave activity on the side of the hemiparesis or sometimes on both sides. The prognosis in this acute onset encephalopathy which occurs 7-14 days after intravenous methotrexate is good.

There is, however, a more chronic encephalopathy which occurs in the same group of patients and in which the prognosis is not so good (10). These patients also have received high-dose methotrexate intravenously. None of these patients had received cranial RT because they have normal brains and they are being treated for osteogenic sarcoma or chondrosarcoma with high-dose methotrexate. Some of them are receiving systemic vincristine as well as methotrexate, and the 2 drugs may be synergistically toxic. The predisposing factors are not known, although it appears that the total dose and the duration of methotrexate therapy are important. Unlike the acute encephalopathy, if one continues to treat these patients, they get worse. There usually is a little bit of improvement after the drug is discontinued, although all of the patients are left with neurological sequelae.

The patients with the chronic type of encephalopathy are mainly children, and most have osteogenic sarcoma, fibrosarcoma or chondro-sarcoma, almost all of them with metastatic disease. The median duration of methotrexate treatment in these patients was 4.3 months before symptoms developed. They had had approximately 11 doses of the treatment at the time the symptoms developed. The dose range was about 8-20 grams/m^2. The drug, of course, in small amounts usually does not cross the blood-brain barrier significantly, but in these large doses there is no question that a great deal of it gets into the brain.

Allen described 7 patients with the chronic encephalopathy (10). Several of his patients presented with personality changes; 2 of them had focal seizures, and 3 had focal signs, usually hemiparesis. Later on, all 7 of the patients became demented and all 7 developed quadri-paresis; 4 of them actually became stuporous. Personality change is thus the earliest sign, with frank dementia later. When the drugs were stopped, many of these patients improved, but all were left with significant residual neurological signs.

The CT scans in these patients can be normal early or show diffuse white matter hypodensity or cerebral atrophy. Later the scans are all abnormal. In 5 patients who had later scans 3-12 months after the clinical diagnosis was made, the CT scans were no longer normal. Four of them showed white matter hypodensity and one of them a focal hypodense lesion. So at the time you clinically suspect a diagnosis by a personality change in an otherwise normal patient being treated with high-dose methotrexate, the CT scan may not be helpful. Later on, the CT scan will show the diffuse hypodensity of white matter and one sees the characteristic changes of methotrexate leukoencephalo-pathy which have been described in the leukemic patients and the others whose central nervous systems have been irradiated.

CONCLUSIONS

The neurologist is faced with a dilemma. It would appear from our experience with systemic cancer that the future of effective treatment of CNS tumors, whether they be primary or metastatic, rests with the use of ever more effective chemotherapeutic agents, probably using multiple drugs in high doses. I think the evidence with primary brain tumors that chemotherapy is an effective modality is now pretty well established. But, on the other hand, the CNS appears peculiarly susceptible to the development of severe and irreversible damage with some chemotherapeutic agents, and the neurologist must watch out not only for drugs which will effectively treat tumors within the CNS but must keep a constant watch on systemic chemotherapeutic agents which may have severe neurotoxicity.

REFERENCES

1. Walker, MD et al, Evaluation of BCNU and/or radiotherapy in the treatment of anaplastic gliomas. J Neurosurg 49: 333-343, 1978

2. Shapiro, WR, Chemotherapy of nervous system neoplasms, In: Primary Intracranial Neoplasms, SHER JH and Ford DH (eds.), New York, Spectrum, 125-140, 1979

3. Ushio, Y, NL Chernik, WR Shapiro and JB Posner, Metastatic tumor of the brain: development of an experimental model. Ann Neurol 2: 20-29, 1977

4. Blasberg, R and C Patlak, Metastatic brain tumors: local blood flow and capillary permeability. Neurol 29: 547, 1979

5. Rapoport, SI, Blood-Brain Barrier in Physiology and Medicine. New York, Raven Press, 1976

6. Neuwelt, EA; EP Frenkel, S Hill, P Barnett et al, Osmotic blood-brain barrier disruption: computerized tomographic monitoring of chemotherapeutic agent delivery. Ann Neurol 6: 166, 1979

7. Hasegawa, H, JC Allen, BM Mehta, WR Shapiro and JB Posner, Enhancement of CNS penetration of methotrexate by hyperosmolar intracarotid mannitol or carcinomatous meningitis. Neurol 29: 1280-1286, 1979

8. Allen, JC, H Hasegawa, BM Mehta, WR Shapiro and JB Posner, Influence of intracarotid mannitol on intracerebral methotrexate concentrations surrounding experimental brain tumors. Ann Neurol 6: 183, 1979

9. Shapiro, WR, NL Chernik and JB Posner, Necrotizing encephalopathy following intraventricular instillation of methotrexate. Arch Neurol 28: 96-102, 1973

10. Allen, JC, G Rosen, BM Mehta and B Horten, Leukoencephalopathy following high-dose intravenous methotrexate chemotherapy with citrovorum factor rescue. Ann Neurol 6: 173, 1979

11. Allen, JC, and G Rosen, Transient cerebral dysfunction following chemotherapy for osteogenic sarcoma. Ann Neurol 3: 441, 1978

13. SUPERIMPOSED VIRAL INFECTION
The Behaviour of Herpesviruses in Immunosuppressed Patients

B. Juel-Jensen

The problem of infection in patients whom you have done your
best to treat for neoplastic disease affecting the nervous
system is a very real one as in any form of intensive treatment of cancer in other parts of the body. The title is
somewhat misleading. The patient who has been treated with
radiotherapy or with cytoxic drugs is not at risk so much
from viruses he meets in his environment, as from those that
are latent in him. You are all well aware of the hazards
the patient runs from bacterial infection that originates
in the flora he normally carries on his skin, in his nose,
etc., a risk which probably is much greater than that of
infection from the environment. I have chosen to say a few
words about the behaviour of herpesviruses in the immunosuppressed patient, for this group of viruses may cause you
the greatest trouble.

May I just remind you that there are four commonly
found in man: herpes simplex virus (HSV), varicella zoster
virus (VZ), cytomegalovirus (CMV) and Epstein-Barr virus
(EBV). Though the behaviour of each of the four viruses is
different in detail, the general natural history is the same.
Each is characterized by a primary infection in the 'non-
immune' host, an infection that may be quite severe but
rarely kills. In the case of HSV the usual site is in the
mouth, as gingivo-stomatitis, although the primary infection
may be of a finger, the herpetic whitlow, or of the eye, or
very rarely as generalized disease, unless it occurs in the
newborn, where the mother has, usually a type II, HSV infection. The primary VZ infection is of course chickenpox,
usually so trivial that most people do not remember having

had it, although nearly everybody has. Likewise, the primary infection in CMV usually goes unnoticed, and it is only
when the immune mechanisms are disturbed that the presence
of the latent virus is obvious. EBV manifests itself as
infectious mononucleosis and although there can be no doubt
that the virus may get reactivated in patients who develop
malignancy of the lymphatic system, it probably does not
give rise to much trouble. All four are very common infections and therefore very important for all your patients.
Speculations have been plentiful as to why these four viruses remain latent and do not recur in most individuals. Although HSV antibody for instance can be demonstrated in a
high proportion of the population, only about 1 in 3 of
those who are herpetic get recurrent lesions. Practically
everybody has had chickenpox but recurrences usually happen
only once, in the form of shingles and usually only after
many years. Cytomegalovirus may never recur in ordinary
circumstances.

We do not know why the latent virus recurs in some
people and not in others. There is no doubt that lymphopro-
liferative disorders such as Hodgkin's disease, multiple
myeloma, lymphatic leukaemia and other reticuloses in them-
selves may give rise to reactivation of the latent virus.
However, treatment (that includes vigorous treatment with
cytotoxic drugs or other immunosuppressive drugs such as
steroids and treatment with deep X-ray) may sufficiently
impair the lymphatic system to cause reactivation of the
virus. Immunosuppressive drugs are used also in patients
who have received an organ transplant, most commonly a renal
transplant. Reactivation of any of the herpesviruses may
imperil the future of the graft, and a very good example of
this is the renal transplant, where cytomegalovirus is
particularly feared (1). Where the patient perhaps in the
past had trivial recurrences of cold sores the institution
of treatment for malignancy may cause a recurrence of un-
precedented severity. An example is a woman in her sixties
who when given large doses of prednisolone suddenly developped widespread ulcerating lesions in her mouth and oesophagus and a dense pneumonitis. VZ virus may likewise be

reactivated and the patient may get repeated attacks of zoster or of generalized chickenpox. Malignancy may be associated with immune complex complications. Purpura fulminans (2) is one such where large areas of skin and deeper tissues may necrotize because of destruction of small blood vessels. Skin grafting may be necessary if the patient survives, unless the virus can be killed.

To the clinician this state of affairs is distressing, but what can he do about it? Clearly forewarned is fore-armed. From experience, mainly in patients with lymphopro-liferative disorders we have found that it is well worth while monitoring for the presence of antibody to the human herpesviruses before treatment is instituted. If they are there but disappear, one is very likely to run into trouble with reactivation and generalized spread of the virus. The patient who maintains antibody throughout is much less likely to get severe recurrences of the infection. The question of destroying the diseased organ and substituting another does not yet arise in the nervous system but it is of some interest to note that cytomegalovirus is more likely to harm patients who are CMV negative if they receive a CMV positive kidney, than if they have already been infected with cytomegalovirus in the past. This might be of relevance when it comes to transfusing patients. That undoubtedly will happen in your practice. If, therefore, your patient is CMV negative it would be preferable to give him CMV negative blood.

What can you do once you have got a reactivation of your herpesvirus? Chemotherapy of viral disease in man is a subject that has received much attention but in which little progress has been made over the last twenty years. Fortunately, some of this has happened in the field of herpesviruses. A large number of drugs have been found to be effective in vitro but very few have passed the test of being effective, yet relatively harmless in vivo, let alone in human beings. The metabolism of the DNA virus is so similar to that of the host cell that the risk of incorpo-rating the substance that harms the virus into the hosts cell is considerable.

The earliest drugs to be used were halogenated thymidine derivatives, of which only 5-iodo-2'-deoxyridine (idoxuridine) has been of practical value. It has been used in an anecdotal way in the treatment of HSV encephalitis, but given systematically it is a toxic substance, and there is no good evidence that it makes any difference to the outcome. The only place for idoxuridine is in topical treatment. It is a very insoluble substance and therefore has to be put up in dimethyl sulphoxide (DMSO) which is capable of penetrating the skin. Applied topically it is useful in the treatment of segmental zoster and limited outbreaks of herpes simplex virus recurrences of the skin.

So often in the immunosuppressed patient the infection is generalized and a systemic drug is needed. The first of these to be used was cytosine arabinoside (cytarabine). This drug is easily soluble and will, in most patients, cut down the period of virus shedding quite considerably, if this is monitored from day to day (3).

Cytarabine has unfairly been discredited, largely because of a double-blind trial, carried out very carefully, in patients who already had lymphoproliferative disease. The drug was given continuously and therefore maximum adverse effect was achieved on the bone marrow, when minimum or no effect could have been predicted at those levels against the virus (4). We have found cytarabine a useful drug, provided it is given intravenously in a bolus once a day, with minimal effect on the normal bone marrow. Adenine arabinoside is much less effective _in vitro_ as a herpes simplex virus killer and I would not recommend it in systemic disease, whereas in our hands it has been a most useful drug in generalized varicella zoster. It has the drawback of being fairly insoluble, it is only possible to get about 250 mg into solution in half a litre of fluid at 40° C. The drug is relatively non toxic.

The following table from the work of Bauer and colleagues (5) shows the relative activity against herpes simplex virus of various antiviral drugs where idoxuridine is used as the reference drug. Acyclovir is of the same order of potency as cytarabine.

Table 1 Relative potencies of 9-(2-hydroxyethoxymethyl)guanine and some standard anti-herpes compounds

Compound	ID$_{50}$ (μM)	Potency relative to idoxuridine ($=$ 100)
Phosphonoacetic acid	57.5	1.7
VIa	40	2.5
Vidarabine	16	6
VIb	10.5	9.5
Trifluorothymidine	1.5	67
Idoxuridine	1	100
Cytarabine	0.2	500
Acycloguanosine (I)	0.1	1,000

Schaeffer and Bauer (1978) Nature, 272,584

The constitutional formula a acyclovir is shown below:

ACYCLOVIR

This drug is remarkable for its lack of toxicity in humans. Its effect appears to be limited to HSV and VZ virus infections. A double-blind trial of its use in herpetic keratitis showed unequivocally that it was effective (6) but clinical trials of its systemic use have yet to be carried out (although they have all been planned and are ready to go ahead). Many patients have been treated anecdotally. A typical example is that of a sixteen year old girl who was admitted under my care in March of this year. She had had chickenpox at the age of five. Acute myeloid leukemia was diagnosed in May 1977. She was treated with cytoxic drugs and a remission was induced. She had whole body radiation and a bone marrow transplant from her brother in June 1978. The brother had also had chickenpox. Seven days before admission she developed facial pain and zoster of the right C2 and C3 segments. This was treated with topical 35% idoxuridine in DMSO, with little improvement. She was therefore put on systemic acyclovir 5 mg/kg eight hourly for five days. We noticed a few new lesions during the first twenty four hours of her treatment but none following that, and all the lesions dried up. Her haemoglobin on admission was 13.4 g with a WBC of 4,700 with a normal distribution and a platelet count of 400,000. These figures were not significantly affected nor was there any adverse effect on liver and renal function during or subsequent to the treatment. We had not dared give vidarabine, let alone cytarabine for fear of damaging the obviously sensitive new marrow. If its early promise is proved in double-blind controlled trials, acyclovir will undoubtedly be a valuable addition to our armentarium of drugs for dealing with the complications by virus disease in patients treated for neoplastic conditions.

REFERENCES

1. Betts, R.F. and Hanshaw, J.B., Cytomegalovirus (CMV)
    in the compromised host(s). Ann.Rev.Med. 28:103, 1977
2. Juel-Jensen, B., Severe chickenpox and purpura fulmi-
    nans in zoster treated with vidarabine. J. Antimicro-
    bial Chemotherapy 2:261, 1976
3. Juel-Jensen, B., Effects of cytarabine on virus shed-
    ding in herpes simplex virus infections. J. Antimicro-
    bial Chemotherapy 3,A:125, 1977
4. Stevens, D.A., Jordan, G.W., Waddell, T.F. and Merigan,
    T.C., Adverse effect of cytosine arabinoside on dis-
    seminated zoster in a controlled trial. New Engl J Med
    289:873, 1973
5. Bauer, D.J. and Collins, P., Schaeffer, H.J., Beau-
    champ, L., De Miranda, P. and Elion, G.B., 9 - (2 -
    Hydroxythoxymethyl) guanine activity against viruses
    of the herpes group. Nature 272:583, 1978
6. Jones, B.R., Fison, P.N., Cobo, L.M., Coster, D.J.,
    Thompson, G.M. and Falcon, M.G., Efficacy of acyclo-
    guanosine (Wellcome 348U) against herpes-simplex
    corneal ulcers. Lancet 1:243, 1979

14. CENTRAL NERVOUS SYSTEM METASTASES IN SMALL CELL CARCINOMA OF THE LUNG – A REVIEW

F.R. Hirsch, H.H. Hansen, O.B. Paulson

INTRODUCTION

Small cell anaplastic carcinoma of the lung (SCCL) constitutes 2o-25% of all malignant lung tumours. It is biologically known to be characterized by a number of clinical features which separate it from epidermoid carcinoma, adenocarcinoma and large cell carcinoma of the lung. The tendency of small cell carcinoma to be ectopically active, and to spread very early and widely is among the most typical characteristics (1).

Local treatment modalities such as surgery and/or radiotherapy have therefore been much less effective in the clinical management of small cell carcinoma than in the other cell types of lung cancer. Accordingly the prognosis for this cell type has been exceedingly poor with an overall median survival of 3-4 months, and with long-term survivors being an exception. However, within the last few years considerable progress has been made in the treatment of this disease by the use of intensive combination chemotherapy, resulting in more than 5x prolongation of the median survival (2).
During this period, central nervous system (CNS) metastases have emerged as a specific problem, presumably because most of the active cytostatic compounds are crossing the blood-brain barrier poorly, thereby leaving the CNS as an unprotected reservoir for metastatic seeding.

The present article will give a short review on the latter subject with special reference to the current status in the diagnosis and therapy of CNS metastases.

FREQUENCY AND SITES OF CNS METASTASES

CNS metastases are classified into three major groups: intracranial, leptomeningeal, and spinal metastases, and each group will be
discussed separately in the present article.

A. Intracranial metastases

Neoplastic dissemination intracranially may be epidural, subdural, leptomeningeal and intracerebral. However, until recently, most
of the publications concerned with clinical intracranial metastases do
not specifically separate the locations of the intracranial metastases,
but refer them as "brain metastases". Epidural and subdural metastases
are rare in SCCL (3) and will not be discussed separately in the present article, while intracranial leptomeningeal carcinomatosis will be
discussed separately together with the spinal leptomeningeal involvement.

Reviewing the literature, it appears that 0-16% of the patients
have brain metastases at the time of diagnosis obviously depending on
the selection of the patient series (Table I). During treatment brain
metastases are reported to develop in another 0-32% of the patients.
Most of the clinical brain relapses are associated with extracranial
dissemination of the disease. Thus, in a study of 145 consecutive patients with SCCL treated at the Finsen Institute, preliminary data indicate that 28 patients (19%) develop clinical brain metastases during
treatment. Only seven of these patients (5%) had clinical, isolated
progressive disease located in the brain (26). As observed from Table
II, clinical brain metastases appear to develop more frequently in patients presenting with "localized" disease (i.e. no detectable disease
outside one lung including regional and supraclavicular lymph nodes),
with a frequency of 12% based on 312 patients in 5 studies as compared
with 7% of 287 patients in 4 studies with patients presenting with
"extensive" disease. Two factors might explain this difference. One
might be the prolonged survival for patients presenting with "localized" disease with a subsequently higher risk of development of intracranial dissemination. This postulation was first suggested by Hansen
in a study of 22 patients with SCCL in which 42% of the patients developed brain metastases with a risk of 66% in the patients surviving one
year after treatment start (27). This concept was later supported by
the results from other studies (21,28); e.g. Nugent found in a study of
2oo patients with SCCL the probability of developing a CNS metastasis
increased to a level of 8o% after 2 years (21).

The other factor which might contribute to the explanation of difference in clinically detected brain metastases is that patients with "extensive" disease often have more marked symptoms from the systemic disease, which may mask slight symptoms from intracranial disease and thereby prevent early detection of the brain metastases. The latter suggestion is supported by the results of the autopsy studies analysed below.

At autopsy, the frequency of brain metastases was 42% (range 28-64%) based on analysis of 968 patients from lo different studies (Table III). In two of these studies, the patient series was analysed with regard to the stage of the disease at the time of diagnosis. Among a total of 157 patients, 28% of 75 patients presenting with "localized" disease had a positive brain autopsy as compared with 44% of 82 patients presenting with "extensive" disease (p > o.o5). Among other prognostic features for the development of brain metastases, Burgess et al reported a significantly higher risk in patients less than 7o years old than in patients over that age (28). A age-dependent risk of developing brain metastases evaluated at autopsy was also earlier reported by Halpert et al in a study of 338 patients with lung cancer, including all subtypes. In the latter study, patients over 5o years of age did not experience brain metastases as frequently as those patients below that age (34).

The sites of brain metastases at autopsy are shown in Table IV. Most of the patients with intracranial dissemination of SCCL had multiple neoplastic lesions intracranially (5,35), and the cerebrum is reported to be the most frequent site of metastases (21,36). As noted in Table IV, solitary pituitary metastases are a frequent finding at autopsy observed in 11% of the patients with intracranial metastases.

B. Leptomeningeal carcinomatosis

Leptomeningeal metastases are a rare clinical finding at the time of diagnosis in patients with SCCL. In 2 studies comprising 152 patients, only one patient was reported to have this complication at presentation of disease (37,38).

During the treatment course of SCCL, leptomeningeal carcinomatosis is observed with an increasing frequency with lengthening survival (21), varying from 4%-11% (Table V).

Based on post-mortem examination, diffuse leptomeningeal metastases were found in 28% of the patients studied by Nugent et al, and they were always associated with other intracranial or intraspinal metastatic lesions. In the latter study, it was of interest that, especially leptomeningeal carcinomatosis was associated with bone marrow metastases suggesting that several mechanisms might generate CNS metastases in SCCL such as haematogenous spread, extension from marrow through penetrating vessels and extension between leptomeningeal, cerebral and spinal sites (21).

C. Spinal metastases

Spinal cord compression may be due to extradural metastases and/or spinal cord metastases. Clinical evidence of spinal cord compression is reported to develop in about 7% of the patients with SCCL (21), while at post-mortem examination 12% of 173 patients examined were found to have tumour within the spinal cord, most of them involving the overlying leptomeninges (21,32).

SYMPTOMS AND SIGNS

A. Intracranial metastases

Symptoms of intracranial metastases may be divided into two major groups: one consisting of focal neurological symptoms corresponding to the cerebral region invaded by the metastases, while the other consists of diffuse cerebral symptoms.

The focal symptoms most often have the form of deficits such as paresis, speech disturbances, hemianopsia, etc., but in some instances the symptoms are of an irritative nature with focal or generalized epileptic seizures.

The diffuse symptoms are most often headache and/or mental changes, due to varying degrees of intracranial pressure gradient, intracranial mass displacement, intracranial hypertension and/or the presence of multiple intracranial metastases.

In our experience, gait disturbances is by far the most common symptom. Thus in a series of 26 patients with SCCL and intracranial metastases who underwent a detailed neurological examination, we observed that 14 patients (54%) complained of gait disturbances. Next to gait disturbances, the most common symptom was headache, which was the presenting symptoms in 7 patients (27%). In some patients, the headache was of typical "brain tumor-type", arising early in the morning upon awakening and disappearing within a few hours. In most instances, however, the headache was of a more stationary type not characteristic of any specific disease. Five patients complained of various cognitive symptoms, five of visual disturbances, four of speech difficulties and four of nausea. Focal weakness was complained of by three patients, while only two patients gave a history of epileptic attecks, in both cases in the form of motor seizures.

At the neurological examination gait disturbances were observed in 15 of the 26 patients (58%), in lo patients in the form of ataxia. Pathological nystagmus, first-neurone paresis, and ataxia of the extremities were each observed in 8 patients (31%), while visual disturbances such as diplopia and hemianopsia were present in 6 patients (23%). Drowsiness was noted in 5 patients and stupor in 2 patients. Other neurological signs such as affected joint-position sense was only observed in a few patients. Only one patient had venous stases in the ocular fundus, and none had typical papillary oedema (36).

Although pituitary metastases are a frequent finding at postmortem examination in patients with SCCL, they are mostly clinically silent. Thus, none of our patients had symptoms of hypopituitarism or of suprasellar extension with affection of the optic chiasma or hypothalamic affection in the form of diabetes insipidus (26).

B. Leptomeningeal metastases

Leptomeningeal spread of the neoplastic disease may involve both spinal and intracranial structures. The symptoms can be divided into three groups: symptoms from the spinal nerve roots, mostly from the anterior; symptoms from the cranial nerves; and symptoms of affections caused by increased intracranial pressure or slight parenchymatous involvement. The latter group of symptoms may be in the form of headache, nausea, gait disturbances and/or extensive plantar response. Major focal neurological deficits are usually not present.
If two of the symptom groups are present, leptomeningeal carcinomatosis is also likely to be present. However, it should be pointed out that many patients with leptomeningeal carcinomatosis have symptoms only from one group.

C. Spinal metastases

Neither clinical symptoms nor signs can give any clear distinction between intramedullary metastases and the more common extramedullary metastases with secondary medullary compression. In our experience, patients with medullary affection complain most often of gait disturbances and weakness of the legs (4o). In addition, there may be symptoms of sensory disturbances and of affected bladder and bowel functions, especially with urinary retention. When the symptoms

progress, there will soon appear the sharp upper demarcation of the
sensory disturbances. Its level may initially lie several segments below the medullary compression, but with progression it will correspond
to the upper limit of the medullary destruction. Pain located to the
site of the medullary compression is common and is often considered to
be an early sign of neoplastic medullary affections (41). It can, however, be discussed whether the pain is due to the medullary compression per se or to metastatic involvement of the vertebrae. Pain can therefore not be used as the only sign of medullary compression, but its
presence should always request a careful work-up. In some instances
when a metastatic lesion spreads along a nerve root, the pain may be
unilateral. This type of pain gives strong suspicion of a metastatic
lesion which might very well go on to compress the spinal cord. A medullary compression, if untreated, will results in progressing neurological deficits, and the final outcome will be complete loss of motor
power, of sensation and autonomic functions from segments distal from
the site of compression.

DIAGNOSTIC PROCEDURES

A. Intracranial metastases

In patients with suspicion of intracranial metastatic lesions
computer tomography (CT-scan) of the head is today the diagnostic procedure of choice. Metastatic lesions change the X-ray attenuation and
may thus be demonstrated. Brain metastases from lung carcinoma without
regard to histopathological subtyping are reported to appear as low-
-density metastases on CT-scan in contrast to metastases from melanoma,
chorionic carcinoma, etc., which appear as high-density lesions (42).
In many instances, the blood-brain barrier will be broken down in the
area of the metastasis, and in such instances, X-ray contrast material
injected intravenously will diffuse into the metastasis, resulting in
a marked enhancement of the attenuation on CT-scan, which is of major
importance in the diagnosis of intracranial lesions, where plain CT-
-scan gives a questionable result as in cases of small metastatic tumours.
Studies with CT-scan in the diagnosis of brain metastases in patients
with SCCL have until now been reported only sporadically. However, in
18 patients with symptomatic brain metastases including 4 patients with
negative radionucleide brain scan (RBS), CT-scan was positive in all
these patients (21). CT-scan as a screening procedure has also been

evaluated in SCCL, but only to a limited degree. In 16 neurologically asymptomatic patients with SCCL, all having normal RBS and skull radiography, one patient was discovered to have a metastatic tumour on CT--scan with the tumour located in the cerebellum (43).

Radionucleide brain scan (RBS) using isotopes such as ^{99m}Tc--pertechnetate has for many years been a valuable procedure in the diagnosis of intracranial neoplastic dissemination. Among patients with symptoms of brain metastases from SCCL, RBS are reported to be positive in about 9o% (5,35).

In neurologically asymptomatic patients the RBS is reported to be positive in only 4% of a total of 235 patients with SCCL compiled by Bunn et al (35). The diagnostic value of RBS is especially inferior to CT--scan in the diagnosis of lesions located in the posterior fossa and those located near the base of the skull, and therefore RBS is today considered to be the "poor-man's" CT-scan in the diagnosis of brain metastases.

Electro-encephalographic (EEG) abnormalities in patients with symptomatic brain metastases from SCCL are reported to be found in 6o-7o% of the patients (5,35). However, a normal EEG is reported in many patients with positive RBS (21), and based on the non-specificity of EEG in the diagnosis of brain metastases, there is no longer a need for EEG in the diagnosis of intracranial dissemination of SCCL if CT--scan or RBS is available.

Cerebrospinal fluid (CSF) examination as a screening test for brain metastases in neurologically asymptomatic patients with SCCL is of no value as described below in relation to leptomeningeal metastases (21). Even in patients with symptoms of brain metastases, CSF examination is reported to be of little value in the diagnosis of brain metastases as far as spinal protein and malignant cells are concerned. Thus, Bunn et al reported a positive CSF cytology in only 16% of the patients with symptomatic intracranial metastases (35). Increased protein levels are reported to exist in about half of the patients with intracranial metastases (5,35). However, this finding is nonspecific for brain metastases (35).

In order to find new parameters for early detection and monitoring of brain metastases, the observation that SCCL may have an ectopic production of some polypeptide hormones such as ACTH and calcitonin, has been explored in the diagnosis of intracranial metastases. Hansen et al have in a recent study measured the concentration of these hormones in CSF in patients with clinical brain metastases and found a significantly elevated ACTH concentration in CSF as compared with patients without any clinical suspicion of brain metastases. No difference between the groups was observed with regard to concentration of calcitonin in CSF (44). Ongoing studies will indicate whether CSF ACTH measurement can disclose intracranial metastases in asymptomatic patients.

B. Leptomeningeal carcinomatosis

Lumbar puncture (LP) with CSF cytology as a screening procedure for leptomeningeal carcinomatosis in asymptomatic patients is reported to be of minimal value. In a study comprising 56 consecutive asymptomatic patients with SCCL, all patients had a negative CSF examination (21). However, repeated lumbar punctures should be done in patients with clinical suspicion of leptomeningeal carcinomatosis in order to find evidence supporting the diagnosis. One or more of the following abnormalities are most often present in patients with leptomeningeal carcinomatosis: increased opening pressure ($>$ 19o mm H_2O), pleocytosis ($>$ 3/ul), increased protein level ($>$ o.85 mg/loo ml), decreased glucose concentration ($<$ 5o mg/loo ml) and/or the presence of malignant cells. Cytocentrifugation of CSF has been shown to be the preferable method for detection of malignant cells and is today widely used also in the diagnosis of leptomeningeal carcinomatosis from SCCL (21,38). However, only 5o% of the patients with leptomeningeal carcinomatosis from SCCL have malignant cells identified in CSF, even after repeated lumbar punctures (21). Thus, many patients with neoplastic leptomeningeal infiltration have no malignant cells in the CSF, and only some of the above-mentioned CSF abnormalities may be present. It should, however, be pointed out that a complete normal CSF examination is extremely uncommon in patients with leptomeningeal carcinomatosis (45).

Myelography, which will be discussed in relation to spinal cord compression, has, after the introduction of water-soluble contrast medium, been able to demonstrate in some instances minimal meningeal carcinomatosis in patients with SCCL (46).

C. Spinal metastases

Myelography is required for definitive diagnosis of spinal cord compression. Lipid soluble contrast medium, e.g. Pantopaque has been most widely used, but new water soluble contrast material with minimal toxicity have been developed and give possibilities for mye-

lography visualizing the subarachnoidal space in more details. But
lipid soluble contrast materials have also advantages as they will remain in the spinal space and can be used for subsequent visualization
of the subarachnoid space without need of repeated lumbar punctures
with new contrast material injections. At present both types of contrast materials will be used in most of the centers.

In the case of a total stop for the passage of the contrast material
it is often necessary to perform suboccipital as well as lumbar myelography in order to demonstrate both the lower and the upper limits
of the cord compression.

MANAGEMENT OF CNS METASTASES

A. Intracranial metastases

The treatment of clinical brain metastases may be divided into
two major groups: acute and non-acute.

The acute treatment may be requested as soon as the diagnosis
of brain metastases has been made or, in many instances, even before.
Corticosteroid treatment is here of major importance. When rapid symptomatic response is required, water-soluble steroids should be used,
e.g. Dexametasone in doses of 3o mg or more per day. Following the administration of steroids, 6o-75% of the patients have symptomatic improvement as early as after a few hours (47). In the long-term treatment prednisone is to be preferred. However, because of the side effect, the steroids should be reduced to the lowest dosage that relie-
ves symptoms; if possible, discontinued after other treatment modalities have been used and shown to be effective. Anticonvulsive treatment
will be required in some instances in addition to steroid treatment. In
patients with symptoms of severe intracranial hypertension and threa-
tened herniation additional therapy with a hyperosmolar solution such
as Mannitol with artificial hyperventilation or neurosurgical intervention may also be required.

The non-acute treatment may consist in radiotherapy and, in a
few instances, in neurosurgical intervention. Chemotherapy is ordinarily not used in the treatment of brain metastases from SCCL.

Based on the high radiosensivity of SCCL and the multiplicity
of intracranial metastases whole-brain irradiation is today the main-
stay of treatment. Probably the most frequently used dosage schedule is
a total dose of 3ooo rads delivered within 2-3 weeks. However, the dose
and schedule of the radiotherapy vary considerably from 1ooo rads in a

single fraction to 4ooo-5ooo rads divided over 4-5 weeks.

More than 9o% of the patients with symptomatic brain metastases are reported to have symptomatic improvement following the radiotherapy (21). The median survival from the start of CNS treatment is, however, rather poor, only 2-3 months (11,21,25,48). However, some authors have reported survivals for more than 17 months in patients irradiated for brain metastases if systemic disease is under control (21,25). Although, the patients have symptomatic response to specific CNS treatment without any signs of later clinical CNS relapse, about 9o% will have a residual tumour at autopsy (21). However, in the majority of the patients, death is attributable to progressive systemic disease rather than to intracranial metastases (21,49). This is also supported by a prospective autopsy study of 28 patients with histologically verified brain metastases in which all patients, except one, had other extrathoracic metastases at the post-mortem examination (33).

No studies are reported yet comparing the symptomatic effect of whole-brain irradiation with steroids therapy alone in patients with intracranial dissemination of SCCL. Many investigators emphasize that steroids should be given concomitantly with the irradiation for the purpose of reducing symptomatic irradiation oedema, but again no comparative studies of cranial irradiation with or without concomitant steroid therapy are apparently reported in the literature for patients with SCCL having intracranial dissemination.

Surgery is not ordinarily indicated in the treatment of brain metastases from SCCL, mainly for two reasons: the high frequency of multiple metastases intracranially and because only very few patients have clinical, isolated brain metastases, as discussed above, thereby leaving surgery almost for diagnostic purposes.

B. Leptomeningeal carcinomatosis

Mostly a combination of intrathecal chemotherapy, e.g. methotrexate and craniospinal irradiation, has been applied in the treatment of leptomeningeal carcinomatosis from SCCL. Recent studies have included the use of intraventricular administration of chemotherapy via an Ommaye reservoir (21). The latter method results in a better drug distribution, and repeated lumbar punctures are not required. Furthermore, the permanent cannula ensures that the drug always reaches the subarachnoid space. The latter method of drug administration is well tolerated and only minor complications either device related such as cannula misplacing, occlusion, infection and neurological

deficit or drug-induced meningismus, headache, nausea and fever are
reported (5o).

Treatment studies with leptomeningeal carcinomatosis from SCCL
comprise only a small number patients (21,37,38,39). Two of these studies in which intrathecal chemotherapy was applied resulted in a median survival of 75 and 39 days, respectively, after the diagnosis of
leptomeningeal carcinomatosis (21,38). Symptomatic improvement was
achieved in 8o% and 4o% of the patients (21,37).

Two facts might explain the poor prognosis for patients developing leptomeningeal dissemination. One is that almost all patients
with leptomeningeal seeding has dissemination elsewhere. Thus, among
24 patients with leptomeningeal involvement from SCCL at autopsy reported by Nugent et al, none of them had metastases at that location
alone (21). Another important therapeutic fact is that only a very
small fraction of the chemotherapy, even when administred intraventri-
culary, penetrates the brain (51) and parenchymatous invation may
therefore not be affected by the intrathecally applied chemotherapy.
Other approaches such as the use of high-dose MTX are therefore required in the treatment of leptomeningeal carcinomatosis from SCCL
(38).

C. Spinal metastases

For patients with symptoms of spinal cord compression corticosteroid therapy is usually given immediately (52), e.g. Dexametasone
in doses of loo mg per day.

Radiotherapy to the lesion is usually necessary immediately
after the diagnosis is confirmed. A frequently used schedule is a dosage of 4oo rads daily for the first 3 days followed by 2oo rads daily to a total dose of 3ooo-4ooo rads. Using this treatment, ambulation
is achieved in about 5o% of the patients with spinal cord compression
with different primaries (52). In the latter study, which comprised
235 patients with spinal cord compression, no difference in the clinical effect was observed when surgical decompression with subsequent
radiotherapy was compared with radiotherapy alone. Those patients who
were ambulatory at the onset of treatment had the best outcome as only
less that 5% of the paraplegic patients became ambulatory (52). In a
study of lo patients with SCCL, symptomatic improvement was achieved
in 5o% of the patients and a stabilization of the symptoms was achieved in the remaining half of the patients (21). The overall median
survival in the latter study was 4.5 months from the start of therapy.

PROPHYLACTIC THERAPY

The prophylactic therapy for reducing the frequency of CNS metastases from SCCL has hitherto consisted in prophylactic cranial irradiation (PCI) and/or the inclusion in the primary treatment regimens
of cytotoxic agents which have shown a certain degree of penetration
of the blood-brain barrier such as the nitrosoureas.

The question of prophylactic cranial irradiation in SCCL was
raised by Hansen in 1973 (27), and since then numerous non-randomized
and a few randomized studies using PCI have been reported. Based on
554 patients compiled in Table II, only 6% of the patients developed
brain metastases during treatment when PCI was given, compared with
19% of the 765 patients treated without PCI. The lower incidence of
brain metastases for patients receiving PCI compared with those patients treated without PCI seems independent of the presenting stage
of disease (Table II).

Four randomized trials with PCI are summarized in Table VI
including 171 patients receiving PCI and 175 patients in the control
groups. Brain relapse was reported in 12 patients (7%) in the PCI
groups versus 31 patients (18%) in the control groups. In two of the
studies, a significant difference in the frequency of symptomatic brain
relapse was found (15,23), while no difference was observed in the
frequency of brain relapse in the two other studies.
However, the studies are not quite comparable as they differ in several important points. The studies of Jackson et al and Maurer et al
include patients without clinical evidence of brain metastases, independent of the stage of disease extracranially, while the two other
studies only included patients presenting with localized disease. The
time of initiation of the prophylactic therapy is also different from
study to study. However, in both of the studies in which PCI reduced
the frequency of symptomatic brain relapse, the irradiation started
early in the treatment course, as compared with the study of Hansen
et al in which the PCI was started 12 weeks after the initiation of
the chemotherapy. This might explain the lack of difference in clinical brain relapse in the latter study. However, the total dose of
PCI given in the latter study was considerably larger than in the
other studies, being 4ooo rads.
It is important to emphasize that none of the randomized studies with
PCI could demonstrate any difference in the median survival, indenpen-
dent of whether the patients received PCI or not. However, the para-

meter for comparison of survival was in three of the studies the median survival (15,23,24). As only about 3o% of the patients would be
expected to develop clinical brain metastases, a lack of difference in
this parameter cannot yet exclude a benefit of this treatment for subgroups of patients, e.g. patients who achieve a complete remission.

Complications secondary to PCI in patients with SCCL have been
reported to be minimal. Detailed analysis of several haematological
parameters in the peripheral blood during the period of the given PCI
was not performed in the studies analysed, so the question of the mye-
lotoxic effect of PCI causing a decrease of the dosage of the systemic
treatment still remains unanswered. Reversible neurological complications two to four months after the initiation of treatment have been
reported by Johnson et al, consisting of poor attention span, recent
memory loss, action tremor, slurred speech, and myoclonus (53). No
long-term follow-up of patients receiving PCI for SCCL has apparently
not yet been undertaken for the evaluation of neurological complications.

The nitrosourea, CCNU, which is reported to be active as a
single agent in SCCL, is today included in a number of the chemotherapy regimens for this disease. CCNU has been reported to have a certain
degree of penetration of the blood-brain barrier and to produce response in primary brain tumours (54). In a compilation of data by
Bunn et al, the prophylactic effect of including nitrosourea in the
treatment of SCCL was analysed in several studies comprising 253 patients of whom 55 developed CNS metastases (22%), which was identical
with the studies analysed without nitrosourea comprising 33o patients
of whom 74 patients (22%) developed CNS metastases (35).

Based on the increasing frequency of symptomatic meningeal
carcinomatosis, the question of prophylactic therapy, especially for
preventing spinal meningeal involvement, has been raised by Brereton
et al (22). However, this complication represents still at present a
minor clinical problem in patients with SCCL, and no reports have
been published using prophylactic treatment to prevent spinal meningeal involvement.

TABLE I

CLINICAL BRAIN METASTASES IN PATIENTS WITH SMALL CELL ANAPLASTIC CARCINOMA OF THE LUNG

Authors	Initial stage of pts.	Prophylactic brain irradiation?	Total no. pts.	Brain metastases at time of diagnosis %	during therapy %	Comments
Eagan et al, 1974 (4)	Localized+ extensive	No	37	14	21*	*Based on 23 patients with clinical relapse.
Newman & Hansen, 1974 (5)	Localized+ extensive	No	46	9	20	
Nixon et al, 1975 (6)	Localized+ extensive	No	28	4	7	
Holoye et al, 1975 (7)	Localized+ extensive	No	39	-	23	
Abeloff et al, 1976 (8)	Localized+ extensive	No	43	8*	18	*Based on 37 pts.

TABLE I (continued)

						Selection, only pts. eligible for a 6-month follow-up are incl.
Hornback et al, 1976 (9)	Localized+ extensive	Yes	29	-	0	
Choi et al, 1976 (1o)	Localized	No	43	-	3o	
		Yes	15	-	7	
Einhorn et al, 1976 (11)	Localized+ extensive	No	29	14	2o	
Herman et al, 1977 (12)	Localized+ extensive	Yes	17	12	0	
Williams et al, 1977 (13)	Extensive	Yes	25	0	0	
Alexander et al,1977 (14)	Localized+ extensive	No	19	0	32	
Jackson et al, 1977 (15)*	Localized+ extensive	Yes	14	-	0	*Randomized study.
		No	15	-	27	

TABLE I (continued)

Levitt et al, 1978 (16)	Localized Extensive	Yes Yes	15 14	– –	2o 14	*Based on 25o pts. with extensive disease.
Moore et al, 1978 (17)	Localized Extensive	Yes Yes	88 152	– 16*	7 4	
Cox et al, 1978 (18)	Localized+ extensive	Yes No	24 21	– –	17 24	Selection: Only pts. with negative prethe-rapy brain scan incl.
Broder et al, 1978 (19)	Localized	No	42	–	5	
Creech et al, 1979 (2o)*	Localized	Yes	171	–	**2 and 18	* Randomized study. **2% of the pts. receiving prophylactic brain irr. vs. 18% in pts. without. Number of pts. in each group not mentioned.
Nugent et al, 1979 (21)	Localized+ extensive	No	2o9	14	26*	* Metastases in all sites of CNS incl.
Brereton et al, 1979 (22)	Localized+ extensive	Yes	33	–	12	Only pts. with CR are registered.

TABLE I (continued)

Maurer et al, 1980 (23)*	Localized+ extensive	Yes	79	–	4	* Randomized study
		No	84	–	18	
Hansen et al, 1980 (24)*	Localized	Yes	54	–	9	* Randomized study
		No	55	–	13	
Hirsch et al, 1980 (25)	Extensive	No	1o5	9	11	

TABLE II

CLINICAL BRAIN METASTASES IN PATIENTS WITH SMALL CELL ANAPLASTIC CARCINOMA

(SUMMARIZED FROM TABLE I)

INITIAL STAGE	BRAIN METASTASES DURING TREATMENT			REFERENCES
	Total*	With PCI	No PCI	
Localized disease	37/312(12%)	15/172(9%)	22/140(16%)	1o, 16, 17, 19, 24
Extensive disease	19/287(7%)	8/191(4%)	11/96(11%)	13, 16, 17, 25
Localized + extensive disease	125/72o(17%)	11/191(5%)	114/529(21%)	4, 5, 6, 7, 8, 9, 11, 12, 14, 15, 18, 21, 22, 23
Total	181/1319(14%)	34/554(6%)	147/765(19%)	

* Patients presenting with brain metastases are excluded.

TABLE III

BRAIN AUTOPSY IN PATIENTS WITH SMALL CELL CARCINOMA OF THE LUNG.

AUTHORS	YEAR	INITIAL STAGE OF DISEASE			NO. POSITIVE/ NO. AUTOPSIES
		LOCALIZED No.pos./No.perf.	EXTENSIVE No.pos./No.perf.	LOCALIZED+EXTENSIVE No.positive/No.performed	
Line et al (29)	1971	-	-	45/1o8 (42%)	45/1o8 (42%)
Matthews et al (3)	1973	-	-	29/1o2 (28%)	29/1o2 (28%)
Takita et al (30)	1973	-	-	22/77 (29%)	22/77 (29%)
Eagan et al (4)	1974	-	-	5/11 (45%)	5/11 (45%)
Auerbach et al (31)	1975	-	-	81/163 (5o%)	81/163 (5o%)
Martini et al (32)	1977	-	-	4o/88 (45%)	4o/88 (45%)
Burgess et al (28)	1979	-	-	7o/177 (4o%)	7o/177 (4o%)
Nugent et al (21)	1979	-	-	54/85 (64%)	54/85 (64%)
Hirsch et al (25)	1980	1o/46 (22%)	19/51 (37%)	-	29/97 (3o%)
Hirsch, unpubl. (33)		11/29 (38%)	17/31 (55%)	-	28/6o (47%)
Total					4o3/968 (42%)

TABLE IV

SITES OF BRAIN METASTASES IN SCCL
=====================================

INTRACRANIAL	Nugent et al (21) (55 pts.)	Hirsch et al (36) (33 pts.)	Total
Cerebrum, alone	9	9	18 (20%)
Cerebellum, alone	0	4	4 (5%)
Brainstem, alone	-	1	1 (1%)
Pituitary, alone	6	4	1o (11%)
Multiple	4o	15	55 (63%)

160

TABLE V

FREQUENCY OF LEPTOMENINGEAL CARCINOMATOSIS IN PATIENTS WITH SCCL.
==

		Total	CLINICAL LEPTOMENINGEAL CARCINOMATOSIS			
			At time of diagnosis		During treatment	
Authors	Year	no. pts.	No. pts.	(%)	No. pts.	(%)
Brereton et al (37)	1978	58	1	(2)	4	(7)
Bagley et al (39)	1978	52	–	–	3	(6)
Nugent et al (21)	1979	2o9	–	–	8	(4)
Aisner et al (38)	1979	94	0	(0)	1o	(11)
Total		413	1	(1)	25	(6)

TABLE VI

PROPHYLACTIC CRANIAL IRRADIATION (PCI) IN SCCL - RANDOMIZED TRIALS

Authors	Year	Initial stage of pts.	Time for start PCI	Dose (rads)	Total (pts.) No PCI	PCI	Clinical brain relapse (%) No PCI	PCI	Median survival
Jackson et al (15)	1977	Localized+extensive	At onset of therapy	3000	15	14	27*	0*	No difference
Cox et al (18)	1978	Localized	–	2000	21	24	24	17	No difference
Maurer et al (23)	1980	Localized+extensive	At the end of chemotherapy-cycle 2	3000	84	79	18**	4**	No difference
Hansen et al (24)	1980	Localized	12 weeks after start of chemotherapy	4000	55	54	13	9	No difference

* significant difference $p < 0.05$

** significant difference $p < 0.01$

REFERENCES

1. Hansen, H.H., Dombernowsky, P., Hirsch, F.R.: Staging procedures and prognostic features in small cell anaplastic bronchogenic carcinoma. Sem. Oncol. 5: 28o-287, 1978.

2. Hansen, H.H.: Management of lung cancer. Med. Clin. North Am. 61: 979-989, 1977.

3. Matthews, M.J.: Problems in morphology and behaviour of broncho-pulmonary malignancies. In Israel, L., Chahinian, P. (eds.): Lung Cancer: Facts, Problems and Prospects. New York, Academic Press, 23-62, 1976.

4. Eagan, R.T., Maurer, L.H., Jackson Forcier, R. and Tulloh, M.: Small cell carcinoma of the lung: Staging, paraneoplastic syndromes, treatment, and survival. Cancer 33: 527-532, 1974.

5. Newman, S.J. and Hansen, H.H.: Frequency, diagnosis and treatment of brain metastases in 247 consecutive patients with bronchogenic carcinoma. Cancer 33: 492-496, 1974.

6. Nixon, D.W., Carey, R.W., Suit, H.D. and Aisenberg, A.C.: Combination chemotherapy in oat cell carcinoma of the lung. Cancer 36: 867-872, 1975.

7. Holoye, P.Y., Samuels, M.L., Lanzotti, V.J. et al.: Combination chemotherapy and radiation therapy for small cell carcinoma. Chest 67: 675-679, 1975.

8. Abeloff, M.D., Ettinger, D.S., Baylin, S.B. and Hazra, T.: Management of small cell carcinoma of the lung. Therapy, staging and biochemical markers. Cancer 38: 1394-14o1, 1976.

9. Hornback, N.B., Einhorn, L., Shidnia, H., Joe, B.T. et al.: Oat-cell carcinoma of the lung. Early treatment results of combination radiation therapy and chemotherapy. Cancer 37: 2658-2664, 1976.

1o. Choi, C.H. and Carey, R.W.: Small cell anaplastic carcinoma of lung. Reappraisal of current management. Cancer 37: 2651-2657, 1976.

11. Einhorn, L.H., Fee, W.H., Farber, M.O. et al.: Improved chemotherapy for small-cell undifferentiated lung cancer. JAMA 235: 1225-1229, 1976.

12. Herman, T.S., Jones, S.E., McMahon, L.J. et al.: Combination che-
    motherapy with adriamycin and cyclophosphamide (with or without
    radiation therapy) for carcinoma of the lung. Cancer Treat. Rep.
    61: 875-879, 1977.

13. Williams, C., Alexander, M., Glatstein, E.J. and Daniels, J.R.:
    Role of radiation therapy in combination with chemotherapy in
    extensive oat cell carcer of the lung: A randomized study.
    Cancer Treat. Rep. 61: 1427-1431, 1977.

14. Alexander, M., Glatstein, E.J., Gordon, D.S. and Daniels, J.R.:
    Combined modality treatment for oat cell carcinoma of the lung:
    A randomized trial. Cancer Treat. Rep. 61: 1-6, 1977.

15. Jackson, D.V., Richards II, F., Cooper, R. et al.: Prophylactic
    cranial irradiation in small cell carcinoma of the lung. JAMA 237:
    273o-2733, 1977.

16. Levitt, M., Meikle, A., Murray, N. and Weinerman, B.: Oat cell
    carcinoma of the lung: CNS metastases in spite of prophylactic
    brain irradiation. Cancer Treat. Rep. 62: 131-133, 1978.

17. Moore, T.N., Livingston, R., Heilburn, L. et al.: The effective-
    ness of prophylactic brain irradiation in small cell carcinoma of
    the lung. A southwest Oncology group study. Cancer 41: 2149-2153,
    1978.

18. Cox, J.D., Petrovich, Z., Paig, C. and Stanley, K.: Prophylactic
    cranial irradiation in patients with inoperable carcinoma of the
    lung. Cancer 42: 1135-114o, 1978.

19. Broder, L.E., Selwary, O.S., Bagwell, S.P. et al.: A controlled
    clinical trial testing two non-cross resistant chemotherapy regi-
    mens in small cell carcinoma (SCC) of the lung. Proc. Amer.
    Assoc. Cancer Res.19: 71, 1978.

2o. Creech, R.H., Seydel, H.G., Mietlowski, W. et al.: Radiation the-
    rapy and chemotherapy of localized small cell carcinoma of the
    lung. Proc. Amer. Soc. Clin. Oncol.2o: 313, 1979.

21. Nugent, J.L., Bunn, P.A., Matthews, M.J. et al.: CNS metastases
    in small cell bronchogenic carcinoma. Increasing frequency and
    changing pattern with lengthening survival. Cancer 44:333-341,
    1979.

164

22. Brereton, H.D., Kent, C.H. and Johnson, R.E.: Chemotherapy and radiation therapy for small cell carcinoma of the lung: A remedy for past therapeutic failure. In Muggia, F. and Rozencweig, M. (eds.): Lung Cancer: Progress in Therapeutic Research, Raven Press, New York: 575-586, 1979.

23. Maurer, L.H., Tulloh, M., Weiss, R.B. et al.: A randomized combined modality trial in small cell carcinoma of the lung. Cancer 45: 3o-39, 198o.

24. Hansen, H.H., Dombernowsky, P., Hirsch, F.R., Hansen, M. and Rygård, J.: Prophylactic irradiation in bronchogenic small-cell anaplastic carcinoma. A comparative trial of localized versus extensive radiotherapy including prophylactic brain irradiation in patients receiving combination chemotherapy. Cancer, in press.

25. Hirsch, F.R., Hansen, H.H., Paulson, O.B. and Vraa-Jensen, J.: Development of brain metastases in small cell anaplastic carcinoma of the lung. In Kay & Whitehouse (eds.): CNS Complications of Malignant Diseases, The Macmillan Press: 175-185, 198o.

26. Hirsch, F.R., Paulson, O.B. and Hansen, H.H.: Brain metastases in small cell carcinoma of the lung. Eur. J. Clin. Inves. In press.

27. Hansen, H.H.: Should initial treatment of small cell carcinoma include systemic chemotherapy and brain irradiation? Cancer Chemother. Rep. 4: 239-241, 1973.

28. Burgess, R.E., Burgess, V.F. and Dibella, N.J.: Brain metastases in small cell carcinoma of the lung. JAMA 242: 2o82-2o86, 1979.

29. Line, D.H. and Deeley, T.J.: The necropsy findings in carcinoma of the bronchus. Brit. J. Dis. Chest 65: 238-242, 1971.

3o. Takita, H., Brugarolas, A., Marabella, P. et al.: Small cell carcinoma of the lung, Clinicopathological studies. J. Thorac. Cardiovas. Surg. 66: 472-477, 1973.

31. Auerbach, O., Garfinkel, L. and Parks, V.R.: Histologic type of lung cancer in relation to smoking habits, year of diagnosis and sites of metastases. Chest 67: 383-387, 1975.

32. Martini, N., Wittes, R.E., Hilaris, B.S. et al.: Oat cell carcinoma of the lung. Clin. Bull. 5: 144-148, 1975.

33. Hirsch, F.R.: Personal communication.

34. Halpert, B., Erickson, E.E. and Fields, W.S.: Intracranial involvement from carcinoma of the lung. A.M.A. Archives Path. 69: lol-111, 196o.

35. Bunn, P.A., Nugent, J.L. and Matthews, M.J.: Central nervous system metastases in small cell bronchogenic carcinoma. Sem. Oncol. 5: 314-322, 1978.

36. Hirsch, F.R., Paulson, O.B., Hansen, H.H., Vraa-Jensen, J.: Brain metastases in small cell carcinoma of the lung: Clinical and diagnostic features in relation to autopsy. (In prep.)

37. Brereton, H.D., O'Donnell, J.F., Kent, C.H. et al.: Spinal meningeal carcinomatosis in small-cell carcinoma of the lung. Ann. Intern. Med. 88: 517-519, 1978.

38. Aisner, J., Govindan, S., Wiernik, P.H. and Gallagher, R.E.: Meningeal carcinomatosis with small cell carcinoma of lung (SCCL): A clinicopathologic correlation. Proc. Amer. Assoc. Cancer Res. 2o: 228, 1979.

39. Bagley, C.M., Einstein, A., Rudolph, R. and Clarke, E.R.: CVM chemotherapy for small cell lung carcinoma. Proc. Amer. Assoc. Cancer Res. 19: 23o, 1978.

4o: Melgaard, B., Paulson, O.B., Arlien-Søborg, P.: Medullære kompressioner ved metastaserende cancer og maligne systemsygdomme. Ugeskr. Læg. 141: 19o3-19o5, 1979.

41. Posner, J.B.: Neurological complications of systemic cancer. Med. Clin. North. Am. 55: 625-646, 1971.

42. Deck, M.D.F., Messina, A.V. and Sackett, J.F.: Computed tomography in metastatic disease of the brain. Radiology 119: 115-119, 1976.

43. Jacobs, L., Kinkel, W.R., Vincent, R.G.: "Silent" brain metastasis from lung carcinoma determined by computerized tomography. Arch. Neurol. 34: 69o-693, 1977.

44. Hansen, M., Hansen, H.H., Almqvist, S. and Hummer, L.: Cerebrospinal fluid ACTH and calcitonin in patients with CNS metastases from small cell bronchogenic carcinoma. Europ. J. Cancer. In press.

45. Olson, M.E., Chernik, N.I., Posner, J.B.: Infiltration of the leptomeninges by systemic cancer. A clinical and pathologic study. Arch. Neurol. 3o: 122-137, 1974.

46. Paulson, O.B., Nielsen, H. and Brodersen, P.: Meningeal carcino-
    matosis demonstrated by myelography using water soluble contrast
    material. In Kay & Whitehouse (eds.): CNS Complications of Malig-
    nant Diseases, The Macmillan Press: 324-327, 198o.

47. Posner, J.B.: Diagnosis and treatment of metastases to the brain.
    Clin. Bull. 4: 47-57, 1974.

48. Holoye, P.Y., Samuels, M.L., Lanzotti, V.J. et al.: Combination
    chemotherapy and radiation therapy for small cell carcinoma.
    JAMA 237: 1221-1224, 1977.

49. Cox, J.D., Yesner, R., Mietlowski, W. and Petrovich, Z.: Influen-
    ce of cell type on failure pattern after irradiation for locally
    advanced carcinoma of the lung. Cancer 44: 94-98, 1979.

5o. Shapiro, W.R., Young, D.F. and Posner, J.B.: Treatment of lepto-
    meningeal neoplasm with intraventricular methotrexate (MTX) and
    arabinosylcytosine (ara-C). Proc. Amer. Assoc. Cancer Res. 16:
    19o, 1975.

51. Blasberg, R.G., Patlak, C.S. and Shapiro, W.R.: Distribution of
    methotrexate in the cerebrospinal fluid and brain after intraven-
    tricular administration. Cancer Treat. Rep. 61: 633-641, 1977.

52. Gilbert, R.W., Kim, J.H. and Posner, J.B.: Epidural spinal cord
    compression from metastatic tumor: Diagnosis and treatment.
    Ann. Neurol. 3: 4o-51, 1978.

53. Johnson, R.E., Brereton, H.D., Kent, C.H.: Small-cell carcinoma
    of the lung: Attempt to remedy causes of post therapeutic failure.
    Lancet 2: 289-291, 1976.

54. Wasserman, T.H., Slavik, M. and Carter, S.K.: Review of CCNU in
    clinical cancer therapy. Cancer Treat. Rev. 1: 131-151, 1974.

15. CNS-LEUKAEMIA PROPHYLAXIS IN ADULT ACUTE LYMPHOBLASTIC LEUKAEMIA

R. Willemze, A.M. Drenthe-Schonk, J. van Rossum, C. Haanen

Introduction

The prognosis for children with acute lymphoblastic leukaemia (ALL) has improved considerably since the introduction of CNS leukaemia prophylaxis by cranial irradiation and intrathecal administration of methotrexate (Mauer and Simone, 1976; Pinkel, 1979). The incidence of CNS-relapses dropped from 50% to approximately 5% of the children. Little is known about the efficacy of this treatment in adults, in whom CNS relapses are also frequent (Willemze et al., 1975; 1979; Gee et al., 1976; Lister et al., 1978 ., Pavlovsky et al 1973).

Since the recent appearance of reports suggesting that cranial irradiation in combination with cytostatic drugs can lead to brain damage (Paylan-Ramu et al., 1978), considerable attention has been given to other approaches to CNS leukaemia prophylaxis. For the same purpose, we performed a partially retrospective, partially prospective study to compare the results of two kinds of meningeal prophylaxis in adolescent and adult patients with ALL treated in the Leiden University Hospital and the Nijmegen University Hospital.

Material and methods

Eighty-six consecutive patients with acute lymphoblastic leukaemia were admitted to the University Hospitals in Leiden and Nijmegen between January 1970 and December 1978. The diagnosis was based on the findings in bone marrow and peripheral blood smears stained with May-Grünewald-Giemsa, periodic acid Schiff, and Sudan-B-Back.(Hayhoe and Cawley 1972).

The diagnosis CNS leukaemia was established on the basis of
clinical signs as well as the presence of leukaemic cells
in the cerebrospinal fluid (CSF).

The ages of the patients ranged from 14 to 71 years, the
mean and median being 27 and 20 years respectively. The
series comprised 34 females and 52 males. Except for blood
transfusions and antibiotics, none of the patients had
received prior therapy.

Complete remission was defined as a state with a normal
peripheral blood picture, less than 5% lymphoblasts in a
bone marrow of normal cellularity, and a total disappearance
of all clinical signs of leukaemia. All other situations
were considered to represent failure. Relapse was defined
as the reappearance of leukaemic cells in the bone marrow,
peripheral blood and/or cerebrospinal fluid, or any signs
definitely attributable to leukaemia.

Remissions were induced with vincristine, 2 mg once weekly
intravenously, and prednisone, 60 mg daily orally. These
drugs were continued for 6 weeks. If complete remission had
not occurred after 3 weeks, daunorubicin, 60 mg/sq.m or
doxorubicin 25 mg/sq.m was added once weekly intravenously
for 2-3 weeks. This protocol was necessary in 39 cases.

To prevent CNS localization of the leukaemia 35 patients
received cranial irradiation (2400 Rad) combined with 4-6
intrathecal injections of methotrexate (15 mg) after a
complete remission had been achieved.

Twenty-nine patients received 3 intrathecal injections of
methotrexate alone (15 mg) during the remission induction
period followed by repeated intrathecal injections at the
beginning of each reinduction course during the maintenance
therapy period. This was performed by Dr. v. Rossum from
the Neurology outpatient clinic.

Nine patients refused prophylactic treatment. The prophylactic schedule used was mainly depending on the hospital
where the treatment started.

In the majority of the patients maintenance treatment
consisted of a combination of methotrexate, 15 mg/sq.m
weekly and 6-mercaptopurine, 90 mg/sq.m daily, both administered orally, alternated with monthly reinduction

courses (vincristine, prednisone). Two to 3 years of
maintenance therapy was given.

Results

Seventy-three of the 86 patients achieved a complete
remission (85%). The median duration of remission was 15
months. The median survival time for all patients is 27
months, compared with 30 months for patients who achieved
a complete remission, and only 4 months for those who died
before treatment or in whom treatment failed.

Fifty patients had a relapse of the leukaemia between 2
weeks and more than 80 months after achieving a remission.
The first relapse occurred in the bone marrow in 40
patients, in the CNS and/or meninges in 5 patients and
both in the bone marrow and CNS in 5 patients (Table 1).
The relation between sex, age, initial leukocyte count,
duration of remission and survival, and the received prophylaxis is shown in Table 2.

Relatively more patients with high initial blast cell
counts received cranial irradiation combined with intrathecal methotrexate.

In case of a relapse of the leukaemia, remission induction
treatment was reestablished. If a remission was not
achieved other cytostatic drugs were added, such as
L-aspiraginase, cytosine arabinoside and cyclophosphamide.
When a second remission was obtained only occasionally
CNS prophylaxis was given.

A second remission could be obtained in 28 patients (56%).
The survival time after achieving the second remission was
approximately 1 year. Second relapses were seen in 23
patients. Primarily in the bone marrow in 13 patients, in
the CNS in 3 patients, in the CNS and bone marrow in 3
patients, in the testis and bone marrow in 2 patients and
with unknown localizations in 2 patients.

Discussion

Prophylactically, the effect in our series of periodic
intrathecal MTX injections seems fairly similar to the
group treated with cranial irradiation and MTX injections,
but the comparison demands some reservation. In the first

Table 1: Localization of the first relapse of the leukaemia in relation to the CNS-prophylaxis received.

Number of patients	CNS-prophylaxis	First relapse No. patients	Localization 1st relapse		
			CNS	CNS + BM	BM
29	Periodic methotrexate intrathecally injected	17	1	0	16
35	Cranial irradiation + methotrexate intrathecally injected	25	1	4	20
9	None	8	3	1	4
73		50	5	5	40

Table 2: Relation between CNS-prophylaxis received and sex, age, initial leukocyte count, duration of complete remission and survival time.

Schedule	Sex M	Sex F	Age Median/Range	Initial leukocyte count x 10⁹/liter Median	Initial leukocyte count x 10⁹/liter Mean	Duration complete remission Median (months)	Duration survival time Median (months)
Periodic methotrexate intrathecally injected	19	10	20 (14–71)	4.0	29	17	34
Cranial irradiation + methotrexate intra-thecally injected	19	16	20 (14–68)	7.9	46	15	28
None	5	4	21 (14–70)	7.2	27	6	20

place, because this was not a controlled study comparisons between various kinds of treatment are difficult to make. Secondly, in the group treated prophylactically with periodic intrathecal MTX, the initial leukocyte count was lower than in the other group, whereas it is well known that high initial numbers of leukocytes in the peripheral blood are associated with a poor prognosis.

In conclusion

CNS-prophylactic treatment is mandatory in adolescent and adult patients with ALL; in our relatively small group of patients both treatment schedules appeared equally effective. But more controlled information is required on the comparative effectiveness of CNS prophylaxis in acute lymphoblastic leukaemia.

REFERENCES

1. Gee TS, Haghbin M, Dowling MD, Cunningham I, Middleman MP and Clarkson BD, Acute lymphoblastic leukemia in adults and children. Differences in response with similar therapeutic regimens. Cancer 37, 1256-64, 1976.
2. Hayhoe F and Cawley J. Acute leukemia: cellular morphology, cytochemistry and fine sturcture. Clin Haematol 1, 49, 1972.
3. Lister, TA, Whitehouse JMA, Beard MEJ, Brearley RL, Wrigley PFM, Oliver RTD, Freeman JE, Woodruff RK, Malpas JS, Paxton AM and Crowther D.Combination chemotherapy for acute lymphoblastic leukaemia in adults. Br Med J 1, 199-203, 1978.
4. Mauer M and Simone JV.The current status of the treatment of childhood acute lymphoblastic leukemia. Cancer Treatm Rev 3, 17-41, 1976.
5. Paylan-Ramu N, Poplack DG, Pizzo PA, Adornato BT and Di Chiro G Abnormal CT scans of the brain in asymptomic children with ALL after prophylactic treatment of the CNS with radiation and intrathecal chemotherapy. New Engl J Med 298, 815-18, 1978.
6. Pavlovsky S, Eppinger-Helft M and Sackmann Murie F Factors that influence the appearance of central nervous system leukemia. Blood.42, 935
7. Pinkel D The ninth annual David Karnofsky lecture. Treatment of acute lymphocytic leukemia. Cancer 43, 1128-37, 1979.
8. Willemze, R, Hillen H, Hartgrink-Groeneveld CA and Haanen C Treatment of acute lymphoblastic leukemia in adolescents and adults: a retrospective study of 41 patients (1970-1973). Blood 46, 823-34, 1975.
9. Willemze R, Hillen H, den Ottolander GJ, Drenthe-Schonk A, Hartgrink-Groeneveld CA and Haanen C Acute lymphatische leukaemie bij adolescenten en volwassenen: behandelingsresultaten bij 75 patienten in de periode 1970-1977. Ned Tijdschr voor Geneeskunde 123, 1782-87, 1979.

16. ABNORMAL CT SCANS OF THE BRAIN IN CHILDREN WITH ALL: THE ROLE OF INTRAVENOUS MTX THERAPY

A. Postma, A. Jonkers, D.M. Mehta, W.A. Kamps, S.S.N. de Graaf

Twenty-five years ago acute lymfocytic Leukemia in childhood was a fatal disease in most cases.
Administration of the folinic acid antagonist methotrexate
by Farber in 1948 opened up new ways to treatment, and
since unremitting development and intensification of chemotherapy induced considerable improvement of survival.
However, when no specific therapy is directed at the central
nervous system, in about half of the patients remission
will be terminated by primary central nervous system
relapse. Once clinically established, this complication is
very difficult to eradicate and the prognosis is bad. The
introduction of cerebral prophylaxis by Pinkel in 1968
meaned a breakthrough in leukemia treatment. Craniospinal
irradiation or cranial irradiation with intrathecal methotrexate at a time when the number of circulating blasts is
lowest, turned out to be highly effective in prevention of
CNS leukemia.
Today more than 50 % of children with acute leukemia will
attain unmaintained remissions of long duration, maybe cure.
Along with prolonged survival toxic effects are becoming
apparent as a consequence of intensive treatment. In the
growing and developing child irradiation of the brain
means a potential hazard. The use of methotrexate has been
reported to result in several complications that may involve the central nervous system.

Several publications appeared on necrotising encephalopathy following cranial irradiation and methotrexate
therapy. Up to now it is not exactly known whether it is
cranial irradiation or methotrexate administration of some
kind which is responsible.
In the Netherlands children with acute lymphocytic
leukemia are registered and treatment is centralised by
the Dutch Childhood Leukemia Study Group. From 1975 to
1978 treatment for the non high-risk group was randomised
in a trial with two arms A and B. (fig. 1 a en b)
In both groups A and B remission-induction consisted of
weekly administration of vincristin together with daily
prednisone during six weeks, followed by cranial irradiation of 2500 rads and five intrathecal injections of
methotrexate and hydrocortison. Below the age of two
years irradiation dose was reduced. Maintenance therapy
started with 6-mercaptopurine daily and methotrexate
once a week intravenously.
In group A maintenance therapy was given during 5 weeks
and alternated with consolidation periods (vincristin and
prednisone as in induction) during two weeks. In group B
maintenance therapy was given continuously without inter-
ruptions. Total duration of therapy was 24 months. The
only difference between the two arms was a consolidation
period in group A and the continuous maintenance in group
B.

In our hospital a total of 21 patients was treated, 15
according to group A, 6 according to group B.
In group B one patient died precocious of pneumocystis
carinii pneumonia and one had recurrent leukemia, which
caused alteration of treatment. So in this group 4
patients are evaluable, who had identical treatment. This
arm was prematurely stopped because of severe complications. Children in group A had no major neurological
symptoms. In four of these children CT scans were

Fig. 1 a.

GROUP A : 4 PATIENTS

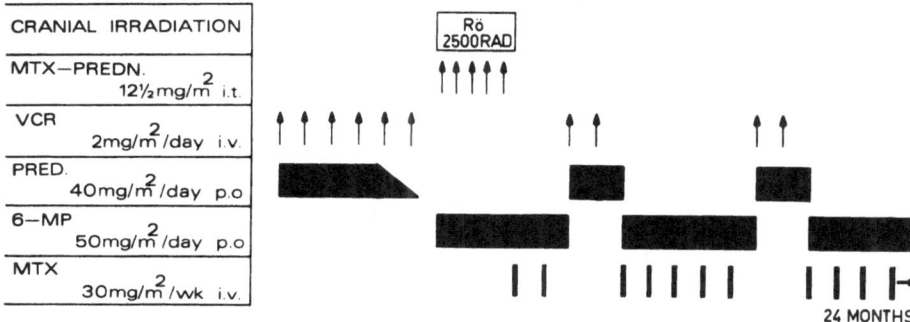

INTERMITTENT MTX
NO CNS LEUKEMIA

Fig. 1 b.

GROUP B : 4 PATIENTS

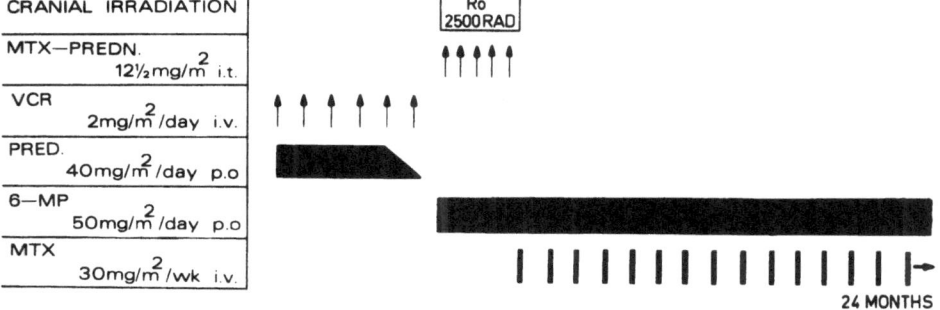

MTX CONTINUOUSLY
NO CNS LEUKEMIA

176

Fig. 2.

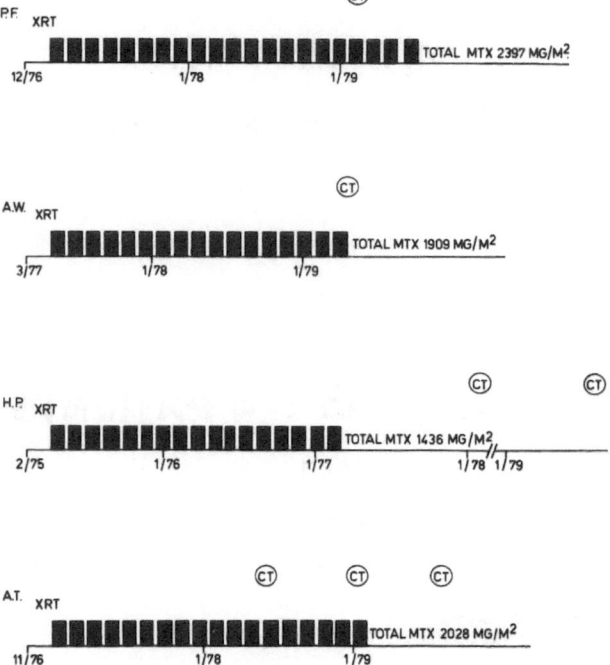

Fig. 3.

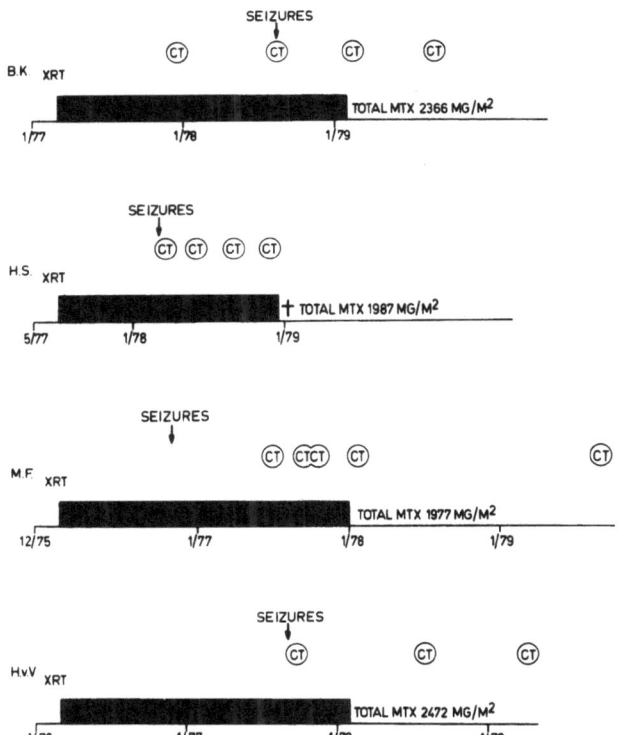

MTX CONTINUOUSLY
NO CNS LEUKEMIA
ALL 4 PATIENTS HAD SEIZURES
ABNORMAL CT SCANS

performed which appeared to be normal. (fig. 2)
All children in group B showed seizures 10 - 19 months
after diagnosis. Examination of spinal fluid in these
children was normal at the time of the first convulsion.
There were no symptoms or laboratory data suggestive for
infectious diseases. (fig. 3)
Computerised tomography of the brain showed calcifications
in basal nuclei and subcortical regions and dilatation
of ventricles. These abnormalities appeared to be
progressive in course of time and even after cessation of
antileukemic therapy. (fig. 4,5,6 and 7)
One of the patients died in an epileptic state. At
autopsy the white matter showed diffuse demyelinisation
and astrocytosis. In the cerebral cortex degenerative
foci with calcifications were found. Virological studies
on this material were negative. There were no remnants of
leukemia.

Another patient in this group who was apparently normal
at time of diagnosis came out with severe mental retardation. So no patient in group A and all patients in group B
showed symptoms of leukoencephalopathy. No CNS leukemia
was demonstrated in any of them. CNS prophylaxis was
carried out according to a standard protocol. The total
doses of methotrexate which were administered were
comparable in both groups. (fig. 2 and fig. 3)

DISCUSSION

The role of methotrexate in the pathogenesis of leukoencephalopathy has been stressed by various authors.
Kay described in 1972 leukoencephalopathy in 7 patients
after long periods of oral methotrexate treatment to
which were added multiple injections intrathecal methotrexate when CNS leukemia occured. When treated with
folinic acid, the deterioration could be arrested and
there had been some improvement. Only one patient

Fig. 4. Calcification in the
cerebellar folia, subcortical
and in the basal ganglia.
Drainage of the hydrocephalus
and subdural hygroma.

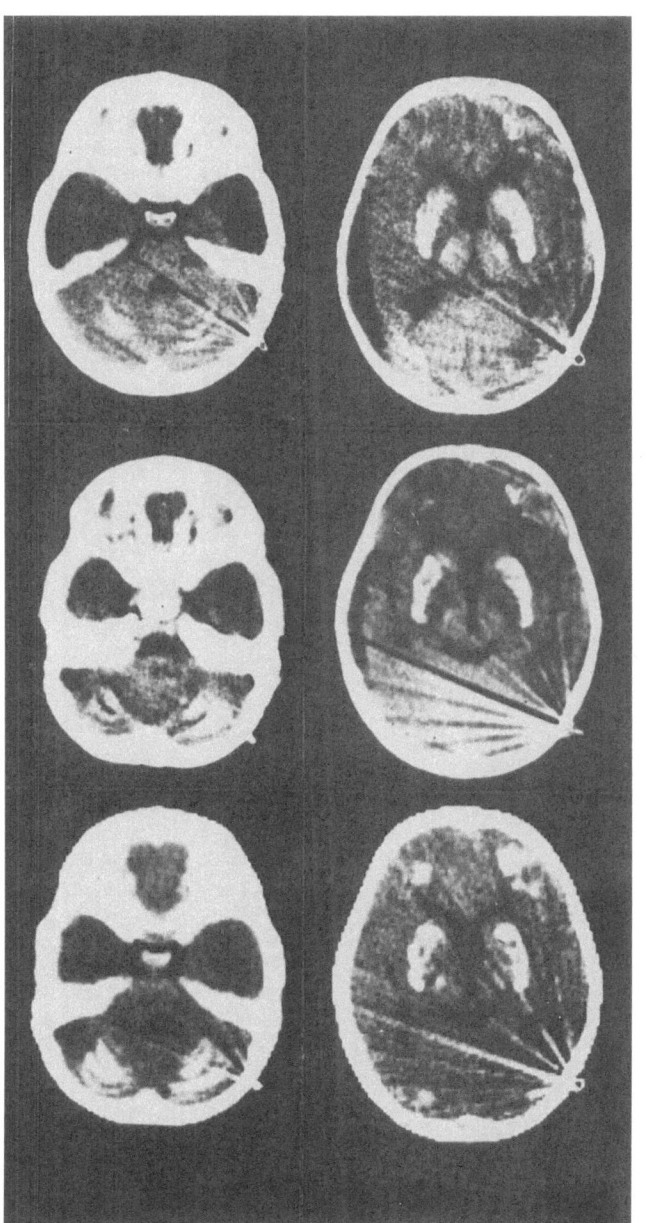

19
months

26
months

44
months

Fig. 5. Developing of hydrocephalus,
        calcification subcortical and
        of the lenticular nucleus.

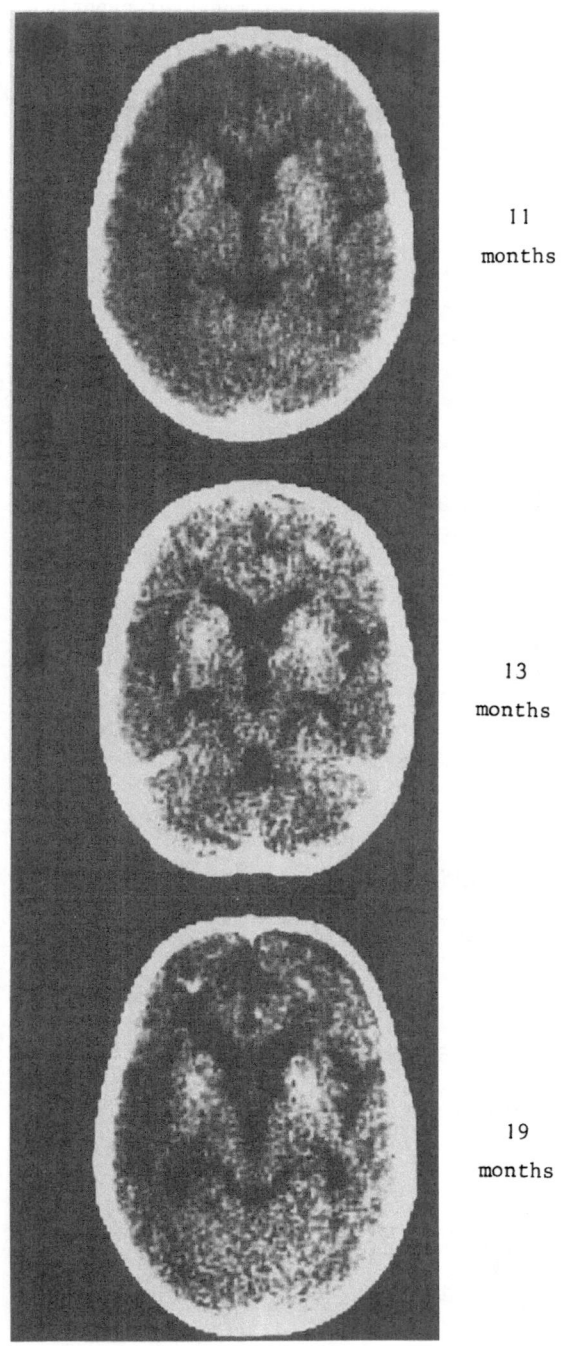

11
months

13
months

19
months

Fig. 6. Calcification subcortical
and of the lenticular nucleus.

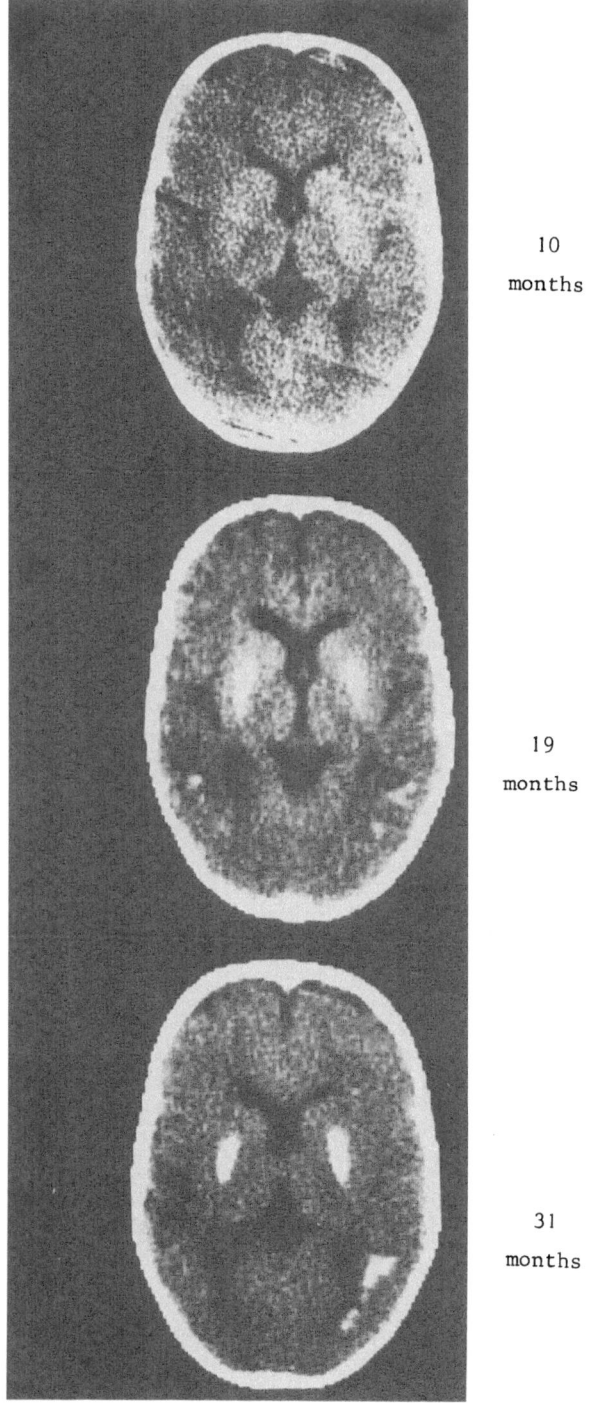

10
months

19
months

31
months

Fig. 7. Subcortical calcification.

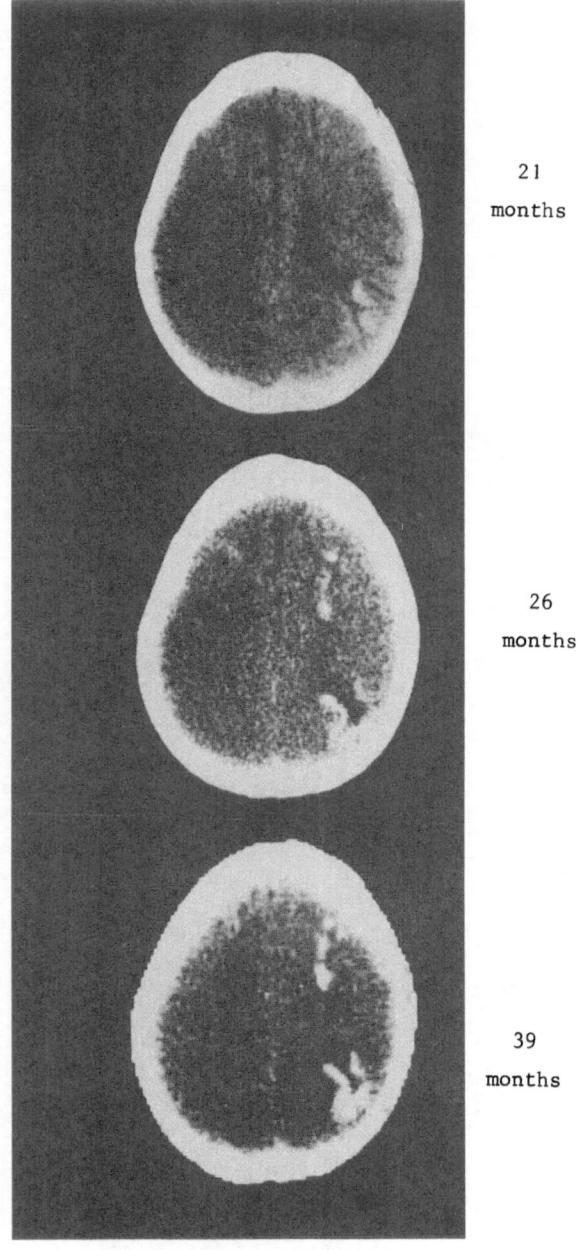

21 months

26 months

39 months

received prophylactic cranial irradiation.
In 1973 Shapiro and Norrell both reported leukoencephalopathy in brain tumor patients after cranial irradiation
and intraventricular instillations of methotrexate. In
the same year McIntosh described seizures and mental
changes following cranial irradiation and intrathecal
methotrexate. Besides her patients received weekly or
biweekly i.v. methotrexate as maintenance therapy;
symptoms diminished after cessation of therapy.
Price described postmortem changes in the brain of
children with acute lymfocytic leukemia; all children
had received i.v. methotrexate after cranial irradiation
with intrathecal methotrexate. On the other hand, no
changes were found in children who had received chemotherapy but no irradiation.

These and other studies share the use of methotrexate,
either intrathecal, intravenous or oral, or in combination.
All mentioned cases had prophylactic cranial irradiation,
except the patients in Kay's study, who were administered
methotrexate by different pathways simultaneously during
prolonged time. Obviously methotrexate therapy is an
instigating factor in the origin of cerebral damage. As
was demonstrated by Whiteside in 1958 the normal blood-
brain barrier is penetrated by small amounts of methotrexate. In mice and cats the blood-brain permeability
experimentally has proven to be increased after cranial
irradiation.
If cranial irradiation in men promotes diffusion of
methotrexate across the blood-brain barrier, then
frequent administration of the drug will effect continuous
exposure of the brain to the drug over a prolonged period
of time.

In our study all patients, who had continuous i.v.
methotrexate maintenance therapy following two and a half
weeks cranial irradiation and five intrathecal injections

methotrexate developed leukoencephalopathy. Patients who
received the same CNS prophylaxis, but maintenance
therapy that was interrupted by consolidation, had no
symptoms. Again the only difference between the two
groups is the whether or not interruption by two weeks
vincristin and prednisone therapy.

In regard to etiology the following assumptions can be
made:

1. The continuous exposure to methotrexate in group B is
   responsible for brain tissue damage.
2. Intermittent administration of methotrexate in group A
   does not evoke brain tissue damage.
3. During intermittent i.v. administration, methotrexate
   in the brain or in the spinal fluid will possibly
   be sustained at lower levels than during continuous
   weekly adninistration, which decreases risk of toxicity
4. Maybe the introduction of prednisone during two weeks
   has protective action against the toxicity of
   methotrexate.

Whichever event may be responsible, administration of i.v.
methotrexate after cranial irradiation carries a potential
risk for severe neurological toxicity which affect
quality of survival.

We think that the weekly administration of intravenous
methotrexate after cranial irradiation and intrathecal
methotrexate induces cerebral damage.

Mr. Chairman,

I showed you one of the most dramatic complications of
leukemia treatment. Nevertheless I do want to stress that
more than 50 % of patients will be cured and enjoy a
good quality of life.

REFERENCES

1. Griffin, T.W., Rasey, J.S. and Bleyer, W.A.
   The effect of photon irradiation on blood-brain
   barrier permeability to methotrexate in mice.
   Cancer 40: 1109 - 1111, 1977.

2. Hustu, H.O., Aur, R.J.A., Verzosa, M.S., Simone, J.V.
   and Pinkel, D., Prevention of central nervous system
   leukemia by irradiation. Cancer 32: 585 - 597, 1973.

3. Kay, H.E.M., Knapton, P.J., O'Sullivan, J.P.,
   Wells, D.G., Harris, R.F., Innes, E.M., Stuart, J.,
   Schwartz, F.C.M. and Thompson, E.N., Encephalopathy
   in acute leukaemia associated with methotrexate
   therapy. Arch. of Dis. in Childh. 47: 344 - 354, 1972.

4. McIntosh, S. and Aspnes, G.T., Encephalopathy
   following CNS prophylaxis in childhood lymphoblastic
   leukemia. Pediatrics 52: 612 - 615, 1973.

5. Norrell, H., Wilson, C.B., Slagel, D.E. and Clark,D.B.,
   Leukoencephalopathy following the administration of
   methotrexate into the cerebrospinal fluid in the
   treatment of primary brain tumors. Cancer 33: 923 -
   932, 1974.

17. PATHOLOGY OF CENTRAL-NERVOUS-SYSTEM DISEASES IN CHILDHOOD LEUKEMIA

R.A. Price

INTRODUCTION

Before the 1950's, the prognosis for children who developed acute lymphocytic leukemia was uniformly poor. Despite therapy that included transfusions and occasionally irradiation to enlarge the viscera and mediastinal masses, 50% of all children who developed this disease died during the first six months following diagnosis and rarely did a child survive beyond nine months (1). Late in the 1940's, Dr. Farber and his associates succeeded in achieving temporary remissions in five children with leukemia by using the folic acid antagonist 4-aminopterol glutamic acid (2). This success lead to the development of more potent antileukemic drugs capable of prolonging initial remissions.

Although early studies showed that extracranial leukemia could be controlled by chemotherapy, meningeal leukemia proved to be more resistant (3, 4, 5). It soon became apparent that treatment of central-nervous-system (CNS) leukemia with cranial radiation of 1500 rads or less provided only temporary gains (6, 7). Attempts to eradicate leukemic cells from the CNS by intrathecal injection of anticancer drugs were similarly unsuccessful (8, 9, 10). From these observations, three points became clear: (i) leukemic cells in the CNS were not as responsive to chemotherapy as were cells in the bone marrow; (ii) meningeal leukemia occurring during remission was usually followed by hematologic relapse, leaving little chance for cure; and (iii) CNS leukemia was one of the main obstacles to successful treatment of acute leukemia in children.

Realizing the high frequency and prognostic importance of CNS leukemia, clinical investigators at St. Jude Children's Research Hospital undertook, in 1962, a series of studies designed to prevent this complication (11, 12). By combining various anticancer drugs and increasing levels of gamma radiation to the central nervous system, they were able to devise a treatment plan that has resulted in remarkable increases in both the frequency and duration of disease-free survival among children with this disease. This innovation in treatment has not been without liabilities: for example, the wider use of cranial radiation to control CNS leukemia has been accompanied by an increase in unusual neurologic abnormalities that cannot be attributed solely to meningeal infiltration by tumor cells (13). The purpose of this paper is to review the main histopathologic features of CNS leukemia and to discuss the pathogenesis of two specific complications of therapy, leukoencephalopathy and mineralizing microangiopathy.

PATHOLOGY OF CNS LEUKEMIA

The four main types of lesions commonly found at autopsy in the brains of children with leukemia are leukemic infiltrations, hemorrhage, infection and complications of therapy. Of these, meningeal leukemia and complications of therapy remain the major concerns of clinical investigators. The frequency of hemorrhage has been significantly reduced as a result of improved methods of treatment. Although sepsis is still the most frequent cause of death in children with leukemia, especially those in relapse, fatal CNS infections account for but a small proportion of the total number of deaths in this childhood cancer.

Information from 100 years of clinical observation and autopsy findings has provided ample evidence that leukemic cells follow a predictable anatomic course as they invade the CNS (13, 14, 15, 16, 17, 18, 19). This pathway is shown in figures 1-3. The first histologic evidence of leukemic cells in the CNS appears in the veins of the meninges covering the surface of the brain. As the infiltration continues, the cells pass through the walls of

188

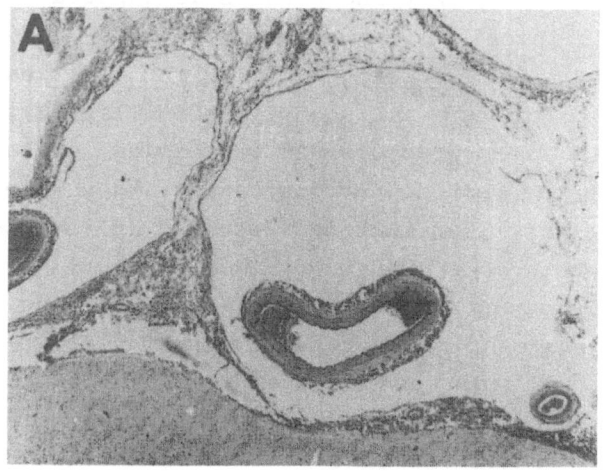

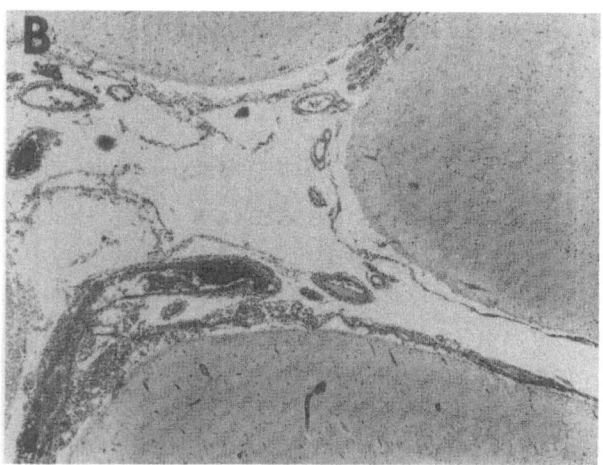

Figure 1: Grade I arachnoid leukemia.
A. Minimal arachnoid trabecular leukemic infiltration and no leukemia in
cerebral spinal fluid channels. Note
infiltrates surrounding normal artery
(Verhoeff's elastic tissue stain, X32).
B. Moderate distortion of trabeculae by
leukemia cells and contamination of CNS
channels. (H&E, X25,6). Courtesy of
Cancer (19).

veins and accumulate in the connective tissues of the arachnoid trabeculae. Afterwards, the trabeculae are destroyed and leukemic cells are shed into the subarachnoid channels, making the cytologic clinical diagnosis of meningeal leukemia possible by examination of the cerebrospinal fluid (16).

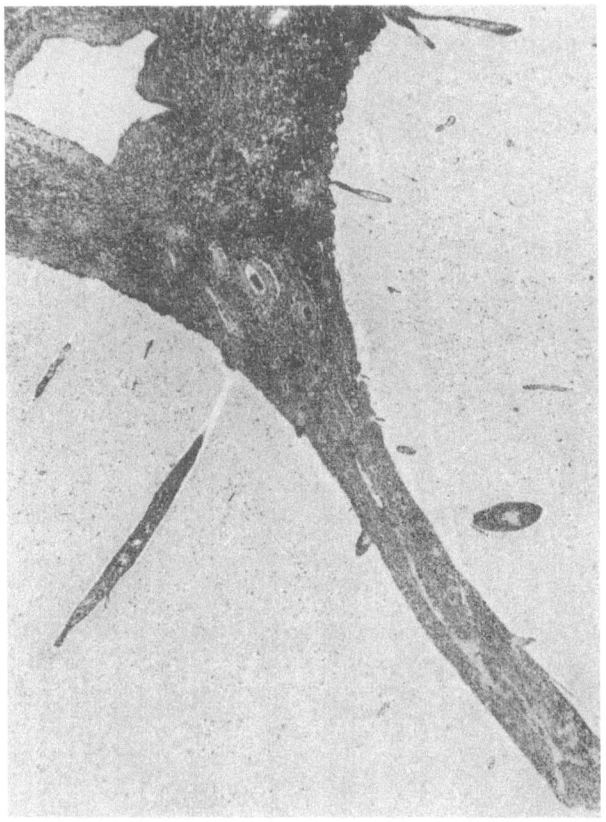

Figure 2: Grade II arachnoid leukemia. Extensive involvement of entire arachnoid with obliteration of CNS channels and compression of small veins. Large vein (upper left) remains patent, but its wall is infiltrated with leukemia (H&E, X26,4). Courtesy of Cancer (19).

As the leukemic cells increase in number, they can be found in the connective tissues surrounding the penetrating vessels in the cortex and white matter. It is important to

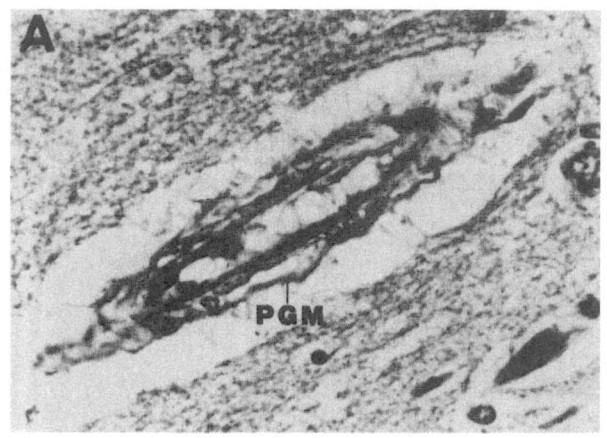

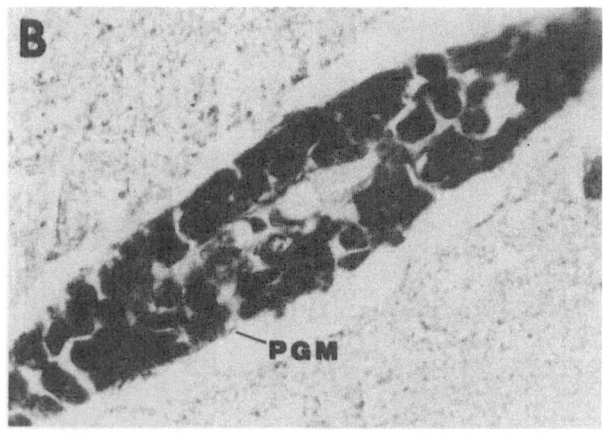

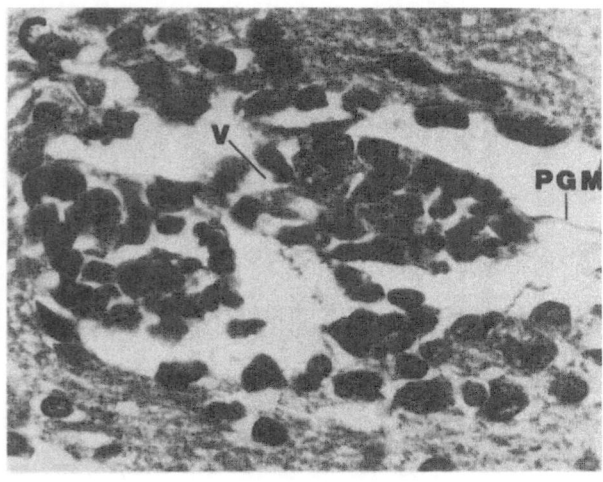

Figure 3: A. Postcapillary venule in cortex with collapsed (fixation arti- fact) arachnoid surrounded by PGM. B. Postcapillary venules surrounded by leukemia cells in deep arachnoid limited by PGM. C. Destruction of PGM at post- capillary venule level and leukemic invasion of adjacent neural tissue. Note absence of hemorrhage and intact venule (V). Gomori-trichrome stain, X680. Courtesy of Cancer (19).

realize that the pia-glial membrane, even at this advanced stage of the disease, separates leukemic cells and CNS neural tissue. Invasion of the neural tissue by leukemic cells occurs only after the pia-glial membrane is destroyed and malignant cells find their way into CNS parenchyma.

COMPLICATIONS OF THERAPY

Finding a completely satisfactory method for treating CNS leukemia has been difficult. Sufficient knowledge about spinal fluid physiology and results of chemotherapy make it reasonable to assume that drugs injected into the lumbar subarachnoid space will reach leukemic cells in the super- ficial meninges over the surface of the brain, but not necessarily those in the deep meningeal tissue (20, 21). Thus, cells in these areas may be left free to proliferate, despite hematologic remission, and eventually lead to clinical relapse. Attempts to diffuse lipid-soluble drugs across the blood-brain barrier and into the brain parenchy- ma would be misdirected, since in most children with CNS leukemia the cells are in the connective tissues of the meninges and not in the neural tissue. Radiation with its ability to penetrate tissues in a uniformly predictable manner eliminates this problem. However, questions naturally arise as to whether this intensified treatment has adverse affects on the CNS. Despite numerous descrip- tions of clinical neurological abnormalities in patients receiving such treatment, histopathologic studies of brain tissue have so far disclosed only two distinctive lesions, leukoencephalopathy and mineralizing microangiopathy (22, 23).

Leukoencephalopathy

The gross and microscopic features of this complication of therapy are shown in figures 4 and 5. Frontoparietal cerebral white matter appears to be most vulnerable while occipital and temporal myelin is usually affected only during the later stages of the disease. Gray matter is characteristically spared in leukoencephalopathy. Marked ventricular enlargement occurs during the later stages of the disease. The principal histopathologic features consist of a multifocal-to-confluent noninflammatory necrosis, occasionally containing mineralized cellular debris, macrophages and reactive astrocytes. Its clinical features include lethargy, ataxia, slurred speech, seizures, abnormal EEG, spasticity, dysphagia, confusion, decerebrate posturing and coma.

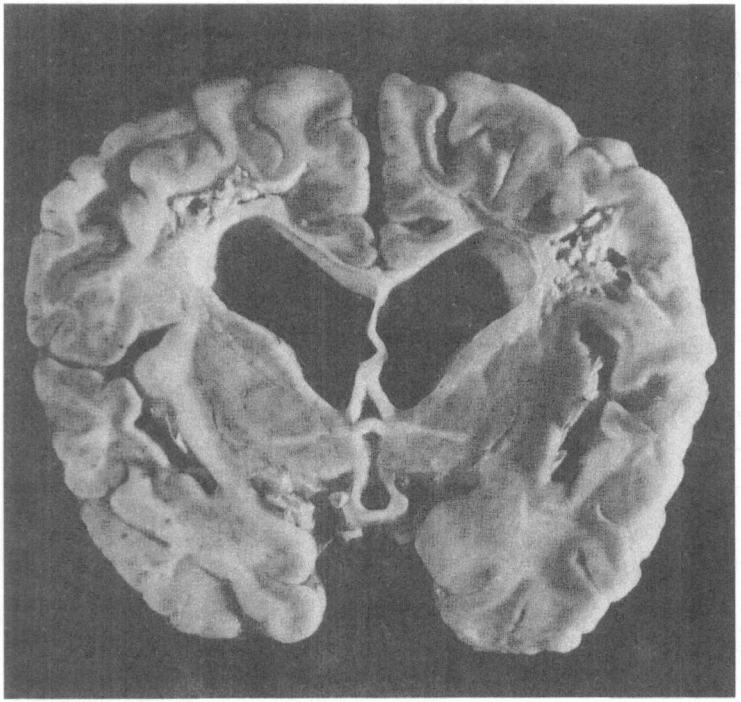

Figure 4: Coronal section of brain demonstrating principal features of advanced leukoencephalopathy. Note enlarged lateral ventricles and necrotic cystic frontal lobe white matter.

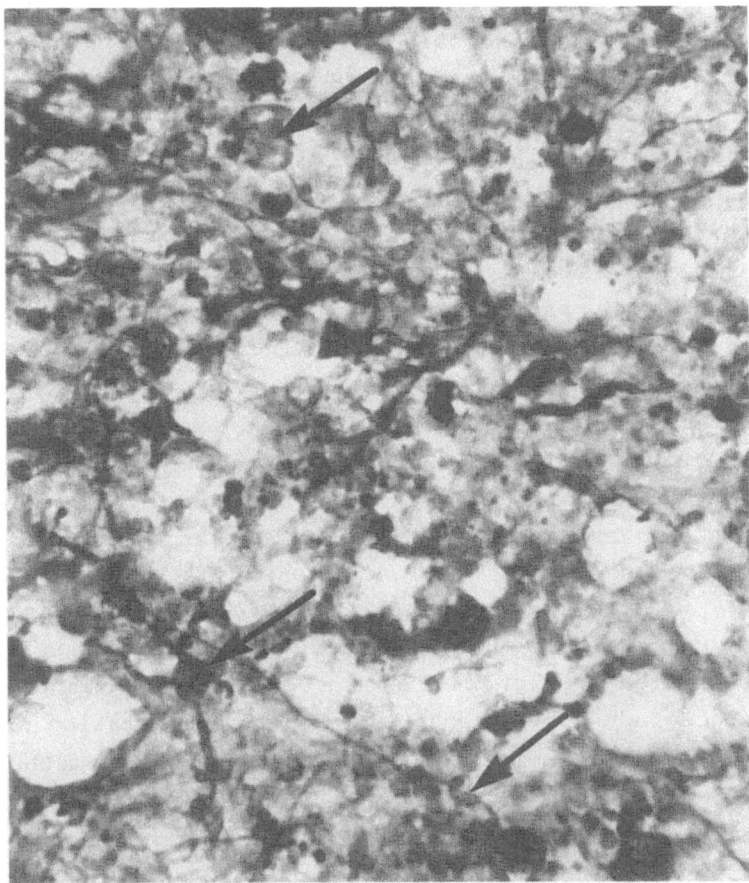

Figure 5: Marked central white matter degeneration and necrosis demonstrating obvious pyknotic and karyorrhectic neuroglial debris and segmental myelin sheath disintegration with characteristic globule and droplet formation. Note focal swellings in myelin sheaths (arrows). (Luxol-fast blue with H&E counterstain, X672). Courtesy of Cancer (22).

Although all factors contributing to the development of this disease are not yet clear, the roles of CNS irradiation and chemotherapy are coming into clearer focus. However, to separate radiation and chemotherapy in any explanation of the pathogenesis of leukoencephalopathy would be difficult based on accumulated knowledge. For instance, although white matter of the brain is more vulnerable to ionizing radiation than gray matter, doses used in the treatment of childhood leukemia are several thousand rads below the levels generally regarded as neurotoxic to CNS myelin (24).

Furthermore, the incrimination of chemotherapy alone cannot be supported by either autopsy or clinical studies (25). Although it may seem attractive to implicate intrathecal methotrexate treatments, it is unlikely that this therapy contributes significantly to the pathogenesis of leukoencephalopathy for reasons which include the following: 1) the flow of CSF carries MTX away from neural tissue, 2) leukoencephalopathy has occurred in children who have not received I.T. MTX, and 3) cerebral cortex and spinal white matter both of which are adjacent to the CSF channels are not affected in cases of leukoencephalopathy (22).

Autopsy findings and clinical observations have provided valuable clues to the cause of this complication of therapy. Children at highest risk to develop the complication are those who have received cranial irradiation of usually 2000 rads or more followed by intravenous methotrexate maintenance given in weekly doses of 50 mg/m^2 or more. A second susceptible group of children are those who receive cranial irradiation in similar doses followed by intravenous methotrexate maintenance weekly in doses limited to 20 mg/m^2 and then develop CNS and hematological relapses, necessitating additional intensive chemotherapy, which occasionally may include second treatments of cranial irradiation (26). Another group at risk are children who receive chemotherapy and radiotherapy of 3500 rads or more for clinically evident meningeal leukemia (27). Leukoencephalopathy has not yet been documented in children with leukemia receiving cranial irradiation followed by oral methotrexate maintenance therapy, nor in adolescents with osteosarcoma being treated with large doses of I.V. MTX, but no CNS radiation (22, 25).

Thus, based on the above information, any explanation of the pathogenesis of leukoencephalopathy must take into account CNS irradiation and methotrexate treatments, since these are the only two factors common to all cases. Furthermore, based on these facts and the well-documented effects of ionizing radiation on the microvasculature, it has been proposed that CNS irradiation damages the blood-brain barrier allowing methotrexate to diffuse into the brain and to cause degeneration of the white matter. This hypothesis is supported by animal studies in which MTX was recovered from the brains of mice that had been treated with 2000 rads of cranial radiation, given in a single fraction, but not from animals pretreated with lower doses or from non-irradiated controls (28). Age at the time of irradiation has not yet been demonstrated to be a factor in the development of this disease. The degree to which meningeal leukemia contributes to the pathogenesis of leukoencephalopathy remains problematic (13, 22, 26).

Mineralizing Microangiopathy

Mineralizing microangiopathy with dystrophic calcification is a second complication of therapy for childhood acute leukemia (23). Whereas leukoencephalopathy affects the telencephalic white matter, mineralizing microangiopathy is confined mainly to gray matter. The increasing number of

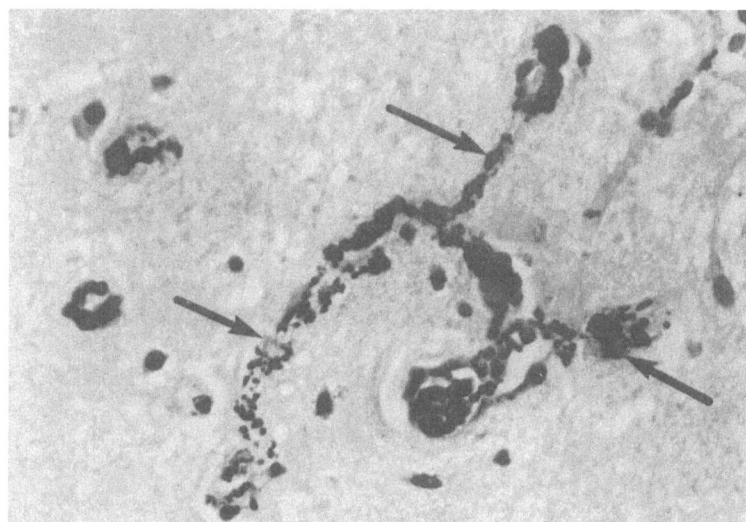

Figure 6: Characteristic accumulation of mineralized droplets (arrows) along distribution of microvasculature (H&E, X310). Courtesy of Cancer (23).

196

reports of children with this disease, and the high frequency with which it is found in brains examined at autopsy, are compelling reasons to assume that mineralizing microangiopathy is the most common complication of CNS therapy in which specific structural abnormalities can be identified (13, 29, 30, 31, 32, 33, 34, 35, 36, 37).

The histopathologic features of this disease consist of noninflammatory mineralizing degeneration of small

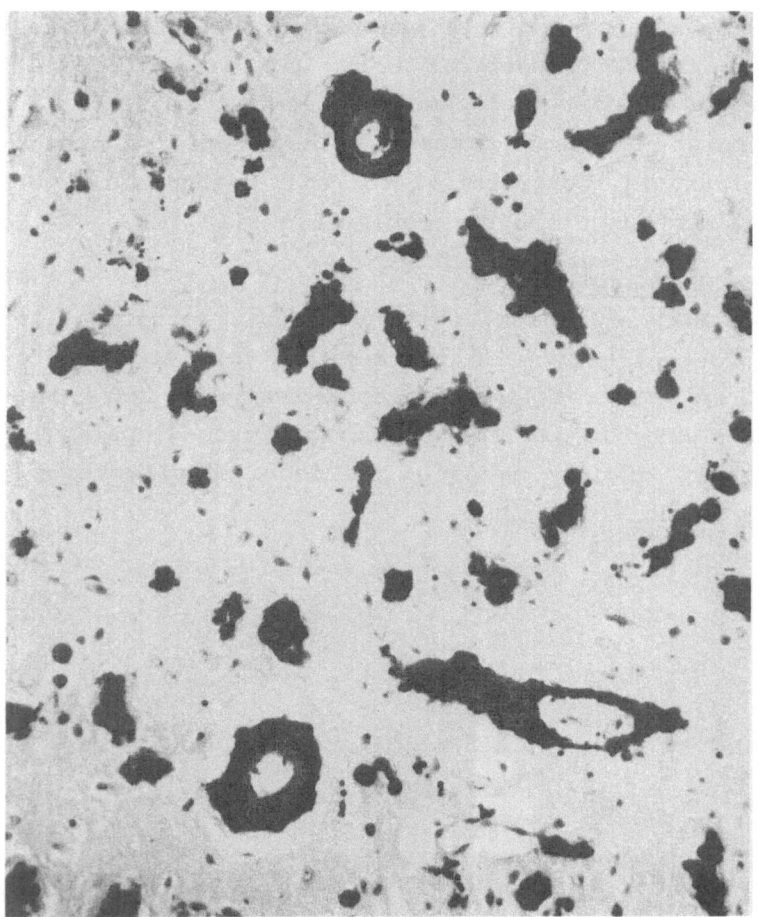

Figure 7: Mineralizing microangiopathy in putamen of lenticular nucleus. Lumens of most smaller vessels are occluded by precipated mineralized debris. Although larger vessels have patent lumens, their walls contain conspicuous amounts of mineralized debris (H&E X170). Courtesy of Cancer (23).

vessels and dystrophic calcification of adjacent brain tissue (23). The earliest histologically detectable stage in the development of the lesion appears as mineralized globules of amorphous material in and around the walls of small blood vessels (figure 6). Advanced lesions contain numerous calcium deposits in neural tissue and laminated mineralized vessels (figure 7).

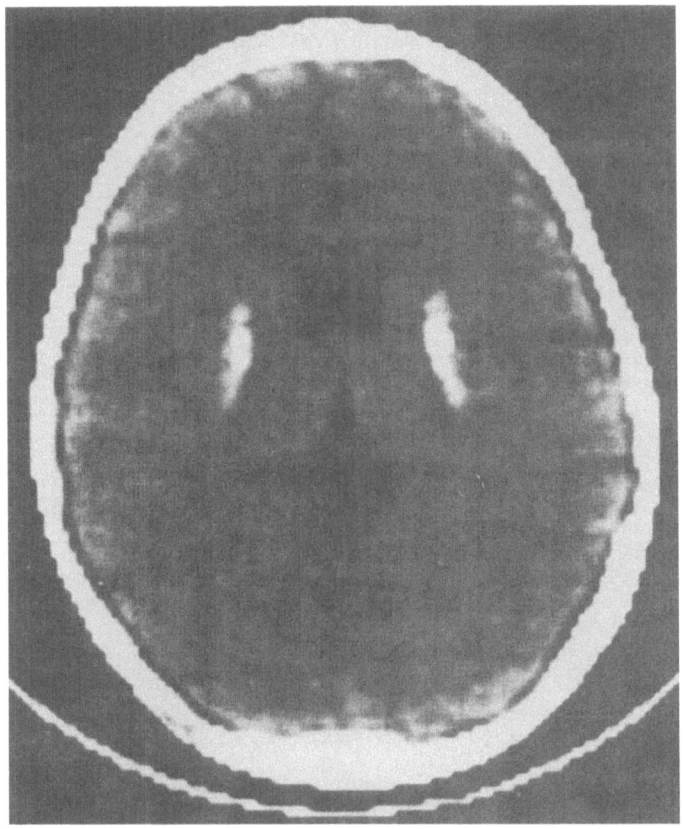

Figure 8: Computed tomography of cerebral hemispheres showing typical bilateral distribution of lesions of mineralizing microangiopathy in putamen nuclei.

A sufficient number of cases have now been studied by autopsy and roentgenography to indicate that the lesions do not occur in a random fashion, but rather appear in specific regions of the brain, generally progressing in a predictable manner (13, 23). With but few exceptions, the disease makes its first appearance in the vascular border zone regions of the brain. Initially, calcifications are

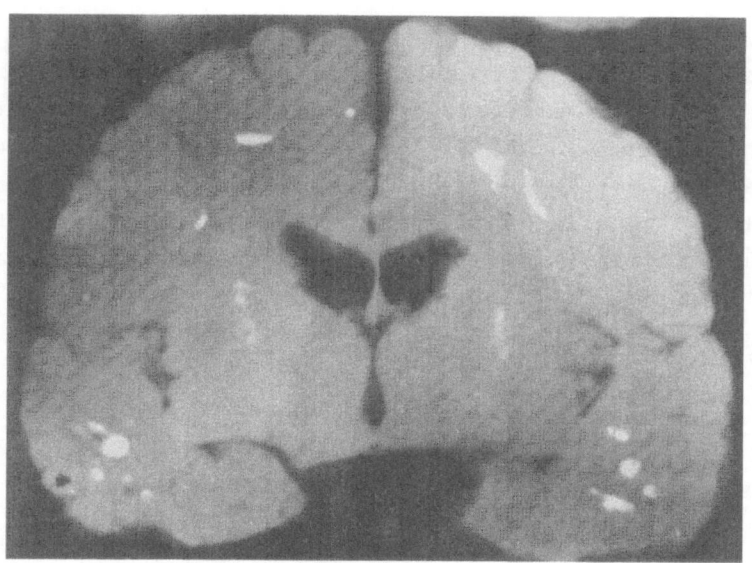

Figure 9: Roentgenograph of coronal section of cerebral hemispheres demonstrating calcified material in putamen nuclei and clusters of similar lesions in the vascular border zones of cortex. Autopsy specimen.

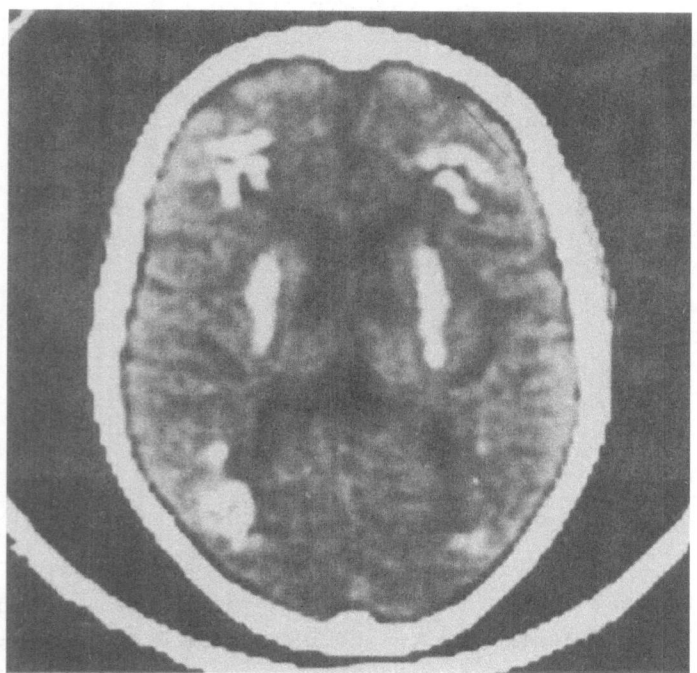

Figure 10: Computed tomography of cerebral hemispheres showing typical bilateral distribution of lesions of mineralizing microangiopathy in putamen nuclei and vascular border zone regions of cortex. Courtesy of American Journal of Pediatric, Hematology/ Oncology (13).

Next, they appear in the border zone areas of cortex between anterior and middle cerebral arteries over the vertex
and middle and posterior cerebral arteries in each occipital and temporal lobe (Figures 9, 10). In advanced cases,
the globus pallidus and cerebellar cortex become calcified
(figure 11). Rarely is the caudate nucleus affected. This
distribution of calcifications produces a characteristic
image on computed tomograms. Thus, the clinical diagnosis
of mineralizing microangiopathy can be easily made on the
basis of striking radiologic findings.

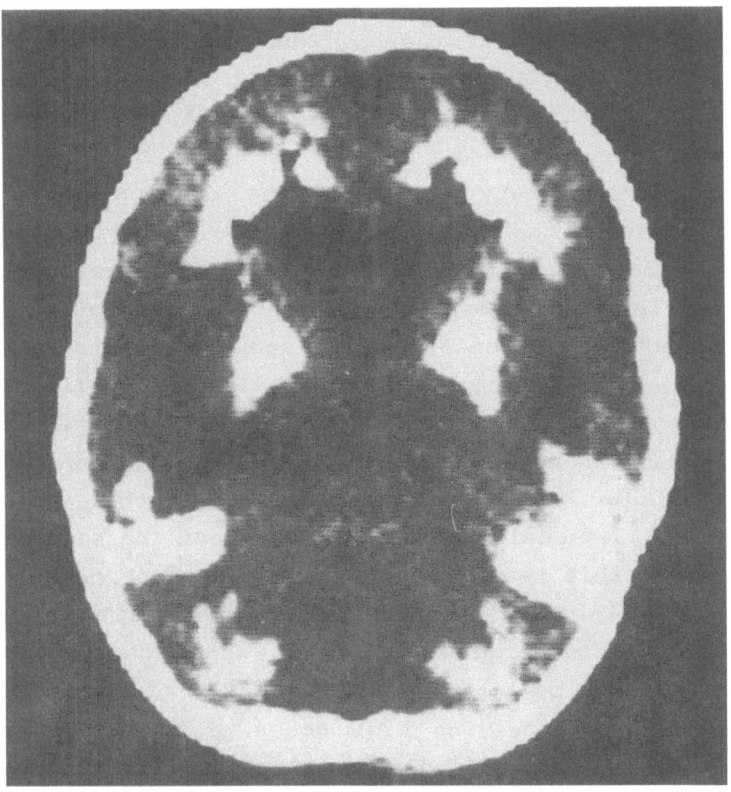

Figure 11: Computed tomographic characteristics of advanced stage of mineralizing microangiopathy. Bilateral opaci-
ties are present in cerebral cortex
border zones. Bilateral cone-shaped
calcifications in center of tomogram
indicate calcification has occurred in
putamen and globus pallidus bilaterally.
Bilateral calcified lesions are present
in cerebellar cortex.

Several clinical variables closely associated with the development of mineralizing microangiopathy have been identified. Children 10 years of age or younger at the time of cranial irradiation are more susceptible to the disease than adolescents (children younger than 6 years are especially vulnerable). The duration of survival is also important (23). If CNS irradiation is the instigating factor in the pathogenesis of mineralizing microangiopathy, then a period of at least 9 to 10 months must usually elapse before either radiologic or histologic evidence of the disease becomes apparent. Another factor that appears to bear on the development of mineralizing microangiopathy is the amount of additional therapy administered for meningeal and hematologic leukemic relapses. The exact contribution of this variable to the development of vascular disease is still undetermined.

How does chemotherapy influence the development of mineralizing microangiopathy? So far, there is no conclusive evidence indicating that methotrexate, the most commonly used antileukemic drug, is the primary cause of this lesion. Although intrathecally administered methotrexate has been implicated in the development of mineralizing microangiopathy (34), there are no convincing clinical or experimental studies to substantiate this contention. If chemotherapy is an important pathogenetic factor, then drugs given intravenously would be the most reasonable candidates, since this route results in the highest concentration of drugs in direct contact with endothelium previously exposed to ionizing irradiation. This concept is supported by results of a study in which 30% of the most susceptible children receiving high doses of methotrexate and cytosine arabinoside developed these calcifications during their initial complete remission following induction and cranial irradiation treatments (36).

Although mineralizing microangiopathy has so far been found only in children with leukemia who have received cranial irradiation and systemic chemotherapy, the exact determinants of its frequency and outcome are not yet known. Many questions remain unanswered. Why are the border zone regions of the cerebral vasculature particularly vulnerable? Once the disease makes its appearance in the basal ganglia, will it inevitably progress to involve the cerebral cortex and cerebellar tissues? Moreover, what determines the rate of this process? What is the incidence of this complication of therapy in surviving children in complete clinical remission following initial induction therapy?

The clinical manifestations of these CNS lesions are still not clear. Despite the frequent lack of congruity between anatomic findings and clinical features in neurologic disorders, a number of neuropsychological abnormalities are emerging with consistency in patients with CNS calcifications (13, 23, 35, 36). The list includes seizures, poor muscular control, ataxia, abnormal EEG, memory deficits, perceptual motor disability and behavioral disorders. Still to be clarified is the relationship of these clinical observations to the progression of the histologic changes of mineralizing microangiopathy and the calcifications that characterize this disease.

CONCLUSION

An understanding of the lesions of the central nervous system in children with leukemia has evolved slowly. Moreover, the pathology of these diseases has changed remarkably since the introduction of effective therapy for central-nervous-system leukemia. In untreated patients, the principle changes were meningeal leukemia and hemorrhage and occasionally infection. Now the neurotoxic effects of central-nervous-system therapy are drawing greater attention than the lesions traditionally associated with meningeal leukemia. It appears that one complication, leukoencephalopathy, can be avoided through the judicious use of methotrexate chemotherapy. The development of the second complication of therapy, mineralizing microangiopathy, may be less dependent upon chemotherapy since it is known that radiation alone can produce microvasculopathy and calcifications in the brain. Only through careful prospective studies can the consequences and incidence of these complications be determined. Information obtained from studies with computed tomography, neuropsychologic examinations, and analysis of chemotherapy will eventually permit sounder judgments as to whether the risk of current modes of CNS therapy for childhood leukemia outweigh the known benefits.

REFERENCES

1. Cooke, JV, Acute leukemia in children. JAMA 101:432-435, 1933
2. Farber, S, LK Diamond, RD Mercer, et al, Temporary remissions in acute leukemia in children produced by folic acid antagonist, 4-aminopteroyl-glutamic acid (aminopterin). N Engl J Med 238:787-793, 1948
3. Sullivan, MP, Intracranial complications of leukemia in children. Pediatrics 20:757-781, 1957
4. Wells, CE, RT Silver, The neurologic manifestations of acute leukemia; a clinical study. Ann Intern Med 46:439-449, 1957
5. Shaw, RW, EW Moore, EJ Freireich, LB Thomas, Meningeal leukemia; a syndrome resulting from increased intracranial pressure in patients with acute leukemia. Neurology 10:823-833, 1960
6. D'Angio, GJ, AE Evans, A Mitus, Roentgen therapy of certain complications of acute leukemia in childhood. Am J Roentgenol 82:541-553, 1959
7. Sullivan, MP, TJ Vietti, DJ Fernbach, et al, Clinical investigations in the treatment of meningeal leukemia; radiation therapy regimens vs. conventional intrathecal methotrexate. Blood 34:301-319, 1969
8. Sansone, G, Pathomorphosis of acute infantile leukemia treated with modern therapeutic agents; "meningoleukemia" and Frolich's obesity. Ann Paediatr 183:3-42, 1954
9. Whiteside, JA, FS Philips, HW Dargeon, JH Burchenal, Intrathecal amethopterin in neurological manifestations of leukemia. Arch Intern Med 101:279-285, 1958
10. Hardisty RM, PM Norman, Meningeal leukemia. Arch Dis Child 42:441-447, 1967
11. Pinkel, D, J Simone, HO Hustu, RJA Aur, Nine year's experience with "Total Therapy" of childhood acute lymphocytic leukemia. Pediatrics 50:246-251, 1972
12. Hustu, HO, RJA Aur, MS Verzosa, et al, Prevention of central nervous system leukemia by irradiation. Cancer 32:585-597, 1973
13. Price, RA, Histopathology of cns leukemia and complications of therapy. Amer J Pediatr Hematol Oncol 1:No.1, 21-30, 1979
14. Fried, BM, Leukemia and the central nervous system; with a review of 30 cases from the literature. Arch Pathol Lab Med 2:23-40, 1926
15. Bass, MH, Leukemia in children with special reference to lesions in the nervous system. Am J Med Sci 162:647-654, 1921
16. Schwab, RS, S Weiss, The neurologic aspect of leukemia. Am J Med Sci 189:766-778, 1935
17. Diamond, IB, Leukemic changes in the brain; a report of 14 cases. Arch Neurol Psychiatr 32:118-142, 1934
18. Leidler, F, WO Russel, The brain in leukemia; a clinicopathologic study of 20 cases with a review of the literature. Arch Pathol 40:14-33, 1945

19. Price, RA, WW Johnson, The central nervous system in childhood leukemia. I. The arachnoid. Cancer 31:520-533, 1973

20. Guyton, AC, The special fluid systems of the body; cerebrospinal, vascular, pleural, pericardial, peritoneal and synovial, In: Textbook of Medical Physiology (2nd ed.). W.B. Saunders, Philadelphia, pp. 72-82, 1961

21. Rieselbach, RE, G Di Chiro, EJ Freireich, DP Rall, Subarachnoid distribution of drugs after lumbar injection. N Engl J Med 267: 1273-1278, 1962

22. Price, RA, PA Jamieson, The central nervous system in childhood leukemia. II. Subacute leukoencephalopathy. Cancer 35:306-318, 1975

23. Price, RA, DA Birdwell, The central nervous system in childhood leukemia. III. Mineralizing microangiopathy and dystrophic calcification. Cancer 42:717-728, 1978

24. Verity, GL, Tissue tolerance - Central nervous system. Radiology 91:1211-1225, 1968

25. Bowles, D, C Pratt, W Evans, RA Price, and T Coburn, Normal computed tomograms of the brain in osteosarcoma patients treated with high-dose methotrexate. Cancer (in press), 1980

26. Aur, RJA, JV Simone, MS Verzosa, et al, Childhood acute leukemia; Study VIII. Cancer 42:2123-2134, 1978

27. Rubinstein, LJ, MM Herman, TF Long, JR Wilbur: Disseminated necrotizing leukoencephalopathy; a complication of treated central nervous system leukemia and lymphoma. Cancer 35: 291-301, 1975

28. Griffin, TW, JS Rasey, and WA Bleyer, The effect of photon irradiation on blood-brain barrier permeability to methotrexate in mice. Cancer 40:1109-1111, 1977

29. Spehl, MJ, R Flament, et al, Diffuse intrathecal calcification appearing during the follow-up of acute lymphoblastic leukemia. Ann Radiol (Paris), 17:417-422, 1974

30. Borns, PF, and LF Rancier, Cerebral calcification in childhood leukemia mimicking Sturge-Weber Syndrome. Am J Roentgenol 122:52-55, 1974

31. Flament-Durand, J, P Ketelbant-Balasse, R Maurus, R Regnier, and M Spehl, Intracerebral calcifications appearing during the course of acute lymphocytic leukemia treated with methotrexate and x-rays. Cancer 35: 319-325, 1975

32. Michotte, Y, J Smeyers-Verbeke, et al: Brain calcification in a case of acute lymphoblastic leukemia. J Neurol Sci 25:145-152, 1975

33. Moir, DH, and PM Bale, Necropsy findings in childhood leukemia, emphasizing enterocolitis and cerebral calcification. Pathology 8:247-258, 1976

34. Mueller, S, W Bell, et al, Cerebral calcifications associated with intrathecal methotrexate therapy in acute lymphocytic leukemia. J Pediatr 88:650-653, 1976

35. Peylan-Ramu, N, DG Poplack, et al, Computer assisted tomography in methotrexate encephalopathy. J Computer-Assisted Tomography 1:216-221, 1977
36. McIntosh, S, DB Fischer, et al, Intracranial calcifications in childhood leukemia; an association with systemic chemotherapy. J Pediatr 91:909-913, 1977
37. Giralt M, JL Gil, et al, Intracerebral calcifications in childhood lymphoblastic leukemia. Acta Haematol 59:193-204, 1978

18. CEREBRO-MENINGEAL COMPLICATIONS IN NON-HODGKIN-LYMPHOMA AND ADULT MYELOID LEUKEMIA

W. Sizoo, J. Holleman

Since it has been appreciated that the cerebro-meningeal sites represent a sanctuary for leukemic cells and require prophylactic anti-leukemic therapy in childhood lymphatic leukemia, the prognosis of this disease has improved enormously. Similarly, cerebro-meningeal infiltration may occur in patients with non-Hodgkin lymphoma and in adult myeloid leukemia, but here the therapeutic implications are still under debate and the value of prophylactic treatment of the central nervous system (CNS) has not been established.

Retrospectively we have analysed the case-histories of 9 patients with CNS complications in non-Hodgkin lymphoma (NHL), in 3 patients with acute myeloid leukemia (AML) and 3 patients with a blastic transformation of chronic myeloid leukemia (CML) between 1977-1979.

In all 15 patients CNS infiltration was confirmed by cytological examination of cerebrospinal fluid (CSF) and/or autopsy. Patients who were suspected of CNS involvement but without proof by histological (pathological) or cytological documentation, were excluded from this study.
In this analysis the following questions were considered:
1. What was the maximal stage of systemic disease throughout its course <u>before</u> CNS involvement and at the time of overt CNS disease?
   What was the time interval between the first diagnosis and the evidence of CNS involvement? Is this predictable?
2. What were the presenting neurological symptoms and findings?
3. Which diagnostic procedures are necessary?
4. What was the response to CNS treatment?

5. What was the survival time after CNS involvement?

1. Stage of disease and time interval

Non-Hodgkin lymphoma (table 1)

Seven of   9   patients with NHL previously had extensive
disease (stage IV) including bone marrow infiltration. Two patients
had only localised disease (stage II) but with subcutaneous lesions
over the skull extending into the bone.

The time interval between the first clinical evidence of systemic
disease and the first signs of CNS complications was highly
variable (range 1-72 months). The clinical status of systemic
disease at the time of CNS involvement is of great interest:
after thorough examination 3 patients seemed to be in complete
remission, while 6 patients showed active systemic disease.

Acute myeloid leukemia and blastic crisis of CML(table 2)

All patients had overt leukemia at the time of CNS disease. In
patients with CML the development into an acute phase of the disease
was diagnosed recently and could not be succesfully controlled by
chemotherapy. From the 3 patients with AML, 1   patient came
initially in a complete remission after 4 months of therapy, but
showed a relapse of the leukemic process 2 weeks after CNS involvement. The other   2   patients achieved only a partial response
  upon   induction therapy.

2. Initial CNS symptoms and findings

In both groups of patients cranial nerve palsies and spinal root
lesions were the most frequent findings (table 3,4,5,6).
Facial nerve palsy was a very obvious symptom and like "spinal root
deficit" it was caused by root infiltration in the area of the exit
from the meninges.
In cases of visual disturbances, reduced visual acuity associated
with an extensive whitish papiloedema, engorged retinal veins and
cotton-wool-like patches on or near the optic disk(see plate 1)

9 Patients with non-Hodgkin Lymfoma,

Previous stage of disease	Time in months until CNS involvement	Clinical status at the time of CNS involvement
IV incl. bone marrow	72	active disease
IV incl. bone marrow	24	complete remission
IV incl. bone marrow	12	complete remission
IV incl. bone marrow	4	active disease
IV incl. bone marrow	3.5	active disease
IV incl. bone marrow	3	active disease
IV + bony skull loc.	24	complete remission
II + bony skull loc,	3	active disease
II + bony skull loc,	1	active disease

table 1

6 Patients with Myeloid Leucaemia,

Original disease	Time until CNS involvement	Status at the time of CNS involvement	Survival after CNS involvement
A.M.L.	24 months	relapse	2 weeks
A.M.L.	8 months	part, rem,	5 months
A.M.L.	4 months	part, rem,	3 months
C.M.L.	72 months	blastic transf,	1 week
C.M.L.	18 months	blastic transf.	1 week
C.M.L.	4 months	blastic transf,	3 weeks

table 2

Frequency of CNS <u>symptoms</u> in
9 patients with non-Hodgkin Lymphoma

Headache	5
Facial nerve palsy	4
Weakness arms/legs	4
Drowsiness	3
Bladder dysfunction	2
Backpain	2
Visual disturbances	2
Deafness	1

table 3

Frequency of CNS <u>findings</u> in
9 patients with non-Hodgkin Lymphoma

Periph. facial nerve palsy	5
Spinal nerve or root deficit	4
Cauda-conus syndrome	1
Cerebellar ataxia	1
Babinski's sign	1
Oculomotorius paresis	1
Optic nerve involvement	1
Retinal infiltration	1

table 4

Frequency of CNS symptoms in
6 patients with myeloid leucaemia

Visual disturbances	3
Headache	2
Weakness of legs	2
Bladder dysfunction	2
Drowsiness	1
Facial nerve palsy	1
Trigeminal neuralgia	1

table 5

Frequency of CNS findings in
6 patients with myeloid leucaemia

Optic nerve involvement	2
Retinal infiltration	1
Protrusio bulbi	1
Spinal cord compression	1
Babinski's sign	1
Spinal root deficit	1
Subcoma	1
Periph. facial nerve palsy	1
Trigeminal neuralgia	1

table 6

Plate 1. Fundus before radiation

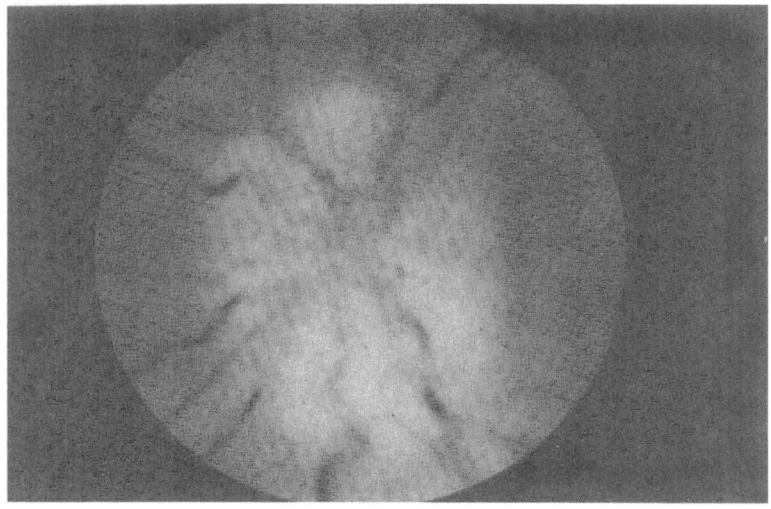

Plate 2. Fundus after radiation

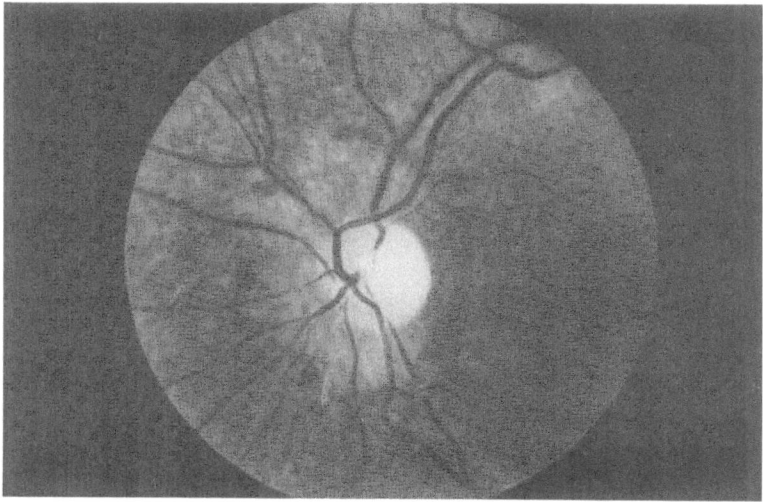

without signs of meningeal irritation, were very suggestive of optic nerve involvement indicating infiltration of the perineural meningeal sheathings and of the optic disk itself. Prompt improvement of the fundus-pathology following irradiation (see plate 2) also points to a local infiltration around the optic nerve.

In general, it is remarkable that the symptoms of meningeal irritation which are frequently seen in childhood lymfatic leukemia, were never noted in these adults.

3. Diagnostic procedures

In 8 of the 9 patients with NHL, CNS involvement was established with the first lumbar puncture by cytological examination of the CSF (obtained by using the cytocentrifugation method). Cell-counts varied from 13/3 cells to 4400/3 cells, all clearly being "non-Hodgkin-lymphoma cells". In patients with AML or blastic crisis of CML, 4 patients had positive CSF cytology at first lumbar puncture, these counts varying from 5/3 (leukemic blasts!) to 700/3 cells. The fifth patient was in a terminal condition and no diagnostic procedures were performed. Autopsy however showed extended cerebral and meningeal blastcell-infiltration. The final patient (CML with blastic crisis) developped over 24-48 hours a spinal cord compression at the level of Th.6, and subsequent laminectomy revealed an epidural manchet of leukemic blast cells from Th.2-Th.6.

4. Treatment, results and survival

In all patients protocol treatment included whole brain irradiation (2500-4000 rads) and twice weekly 15 mg methotrexate, administered intrathecally by lumbar puncture.
Additional spine irradiation was given (to replace intrathecal therapy) only when:
- positive CSF cytology persisted or recurred during intrathecal MTX treatment (1 NHL patient), and/or:
- tumor masses were visible at myelography (2 NHL patients),

- lumbar punctures were associated with technical difficulties
  (1 NHL patient).

In_the_NHL_group_(n=9) (table 7), 4 patients were routinely treated
with brain irradiation + MTX intrathecally. Three of them showed
regression of neurological signs with simultaneously a rapid disappearance of the pathological cells from the CSF; one patients did
not show improvement, though CSF cytology became negative.
Four other patients required additional spinal irradiation for
reasons mentioned above. All of them responded well with a regression of neurological symptoms, though only 3 showed normalisation
of CSF cytology; the fourth patient maintained a positive CSF for
unknown reasons (all cultures being negative).
Finally, 1 patient was started on brain radiation but deteriorated
rapidly and died from generalised symptoms within 1 month.

In conclusion: out of these 9 patients 7 died within 6 months,
evidently not as a result of CNS involvement but all of them from
generalised systemic disease.

In_the_AML_and_CML_group_(n=6) (table 2) the results were even
worse: 4 patients died within 1 month from generalised leukemic
symptoms before CNS treatment was completed. Only 2 patients
finished CNS therapy; their neurological symptoms disappeared and
CSF cytology turned negative. However, also these 2 patients died
from complications of systemic leukemia respectively within 3 and 5
months after evidence of CNS disease.

5. Prognosis

Since of both groups of patients many seem to die relatively soon
after CNS involvement, one might question the necessity of extensive
CNS therapy. We feel that CNS treatment is justified for the
following reasons:
1. Improvement of neurological symptoms to CNS treatment is fast
   and therefore a relief for the patient.
2. The response of systemic disease to chemotherapy for each
   individual is not predictable and hopefully will become better
   in the future.

214

Results of CNS treatment in 9
patients with non-Hodgkin Lymfoma

Treatment	Clinical improvement	CSF cytology after therapy	Survival after CNS involv. in months
W.B.I. + MTX i.th.	good	neg.	6 †
W.B.I. + MTX i.th.	good	neg.	4 †
W.B.I. + MTX i.th.	nihil	neg.	4 †
W.B.I. + MTX i.th.	moderate	neg.	3
W.B.I. + MTX i.th. + spinal radiation	good	neg	7
W.B.I. + MTX i.th. + spinal radiation	moderate	pos.	5 †
W.B.I. + MTX i.th. + spinal radiation	good	neg.	4 †
W.B.I. + MTX i.th. + spinal radiation	good	neg.	1 †
W.B.I.	moderate	?	1 †

Note: all deaths were due to generalised systemic disease
Note: spinal radiation was given when MTX i.th. failed and/or in case of positive myelography.

table 7

3. Lack of CNS treatment means certain neurological death for the
   few patients whose systemic disease will remain under control
   for a long period of time.

A quite serious problem is the neurotoxicity of intrathecal methotrexate consisting of chemical arachnoiditis, paralysis and encephalopathy (table 9). Also other cytostatic agents like ara-C are
notorious for these complications. It is wellknown that in cases of
CNS disease this type of complications is worse than in case of
prophylactic treatment.
Specifically, chemical arachnoiditis with headache, dizziness and
backpain was a very common finding in our patients. However, these
complications did not influence the prognosis of CNS- or systemic
disease.

Conclusions

It is clear that CNS infiltration is a very bad prognostic factor in
myeloid leukemia and to a lesser extent in NHL. Though nearly all
patients responded well to CNS therapy, many of them died rapidly as a
result of progressive systemic disease. Since a similar poor outcome
was seen in some patients who were believed to be in complete clinical
remission at the time of CNS involvement, it may be suggested that
these patients carried subclinically allready a substantial tumor load.
This would mean that CNS relapse in myeloid leukemia and NHL does not
emerge as an isolated relapse like in childhood lymphatic leukemia, but
rather as part of a disseminated recurrence. Therefore under these conditions CNS treatment with an impact on survival is most probably
directly related to succesful control of the tumor elsewhere.
Until now prophylactic treatment of the brain and medulla has not yet
been evaluated systematically. Therefore it remains uncertain whether
CNS disease originates from malignant cells present in a CNS sanctuary
since the first time of diagnosis, or from cells which have seeded into
the CNS at a later stage of the disease following a (clinical or sub-
clinical) relapse elsewhere. If the latter possibility would apply,
prophylactic treatment of the CNS would be useless.
However, since this mechanism is still unknown and moreover because of

Neurotoxic reactions due to intrathecal MTX

Side effects	Incidence	Symptoms or signs
1. Chemical arachnoiditis (meningeal irritation)	Common	back pain, fever, dizziness, neck stiffness, headache, vomiting, CSF pleocytosis

2. Weakness or paralysis
  a. transient
  b. permanent
	Rare	back pain, weakness, paralysis

3. Encephalopathy
  a. transient
  b. progressive or lethal
	Rare	somnolence, coma, dementia ataxia, convulsions, death

table 8

the unfavourable outcome once CNS disease has occurred, there are
valid reasons to try and define the prognostic indications for development of CNS involvement at an early stage of systemic disease, in order
to elaborate the value of CNS prophylaxis.

Since CNS involvement in the whole group of patients with NHL has a
relatively low incidence, it would appear that prophylaxis should not
be applied to áll patients (as in acute lymphocytic leukemia), but only
to suspected high-risk subgroups. Recently it has been suggested that
among the group of non-Hodgkin-Lymphomas specifically patients with
the histological subtype of diffuse histiosarcoma with bone marrow
involvement as one of the initial symptoms, are a serious high risk
group who might benefit from CNS prophylaxis.
In patients with myeloid leukemia the prognosis quod vitam is so very
poor that at this moment prophylactic CNS treatment seems not justi-
fiable.

Acknowledgements
We are grateful to T.C.M. van Woerkom, neurologist, and L.J. de Heer,
ophthalmologist, for their diagnostic help and their advice concerning
these patients.

Dept. of Hematology, Rott.Radio Therapeutical Institute, Rotterdam,

REFERENCES

1. Azzarelli, B, et al, Pathogenesis of Central Nervous System
   Infiltration in Acute Leukemia.
   Arch.Path.Lab.Med., 101: 203-205, 1977.
2. Bunn, P.A., et al, Central Nervous System Complications in Patients
   With Diffuse Histiocytic and Undifferentiated Lymphoma:
   Leukemia Revisited.
   Blood, 47: 3-10, 1976.
3. Dawson, D.M., et al, Neurological Complications of Acute Leukemia
   in Adults: Changing Rate.
   Ann.intern.Med., 79: 541-544, 1973.
4. Herman, T.S., et al, Involvement of the Central Nervous System by
   Non-Hodgkin's Lymphoma.
   Cancer, 43: 390-397, 1979.
5. Law, I.P., et al, Involvement of the Central Nervous System in
   Non-Hodgkin's Lymphoma.
   Cancer, 36: 225-231, 1975.
6. Law, I.P., et al, Adult Central Nervous System Leukemia: Incidence
   and Clinicopathologic Features.
   Sth.med.J., 69: 1054-1057, 1976.
7. Law, I.P., et al, Adult Acute Leukemia: Frequency of Central Nervous
   System Involvement in Long Term Survivors.
   Cancer, 40: 1304-1306, 1977
8. Meyer, R.J., et al, Central Nervous System Involvement at Presentation in the Chronic Phase of Chronic Myelogenous Leukemia in
   Childhood.
   Cancer, 42: 305-310, 1978.
9. Pippard, M.J., et al, Infiltration of Central Nervous System in
   Adult Acute Myeloid Leukaemia.
   Brit.med.J., 1: 227-229, 1979.
10.Pochedly, C, Neurotoxicity Due to CNS Therapy for Leukemia.
   Med.and Pediatr.Oncol., 3: 101-115, 1977.
11.Preston, F.E., et al, Cellular Hyperviscosity as a Cause of Neuro-
   logical Symptoms in Leukaemia.
   Brit.med.J., 1: 476-478, 1978.
12.Reddick, R.L., et al, Immunoblastic Sarcoma of the Central Nervous
   System in a Patient with Lymphomatoid Granulomatosis.
   Cancer, 42: 652-659, 1978.
13.Sweet, D.L., et al, Central Nervous System Involvement in Patients
   With Histiocytic Lymphoma, Diffuse Type.
   Blood, 51: 177-179, 1978.
14.Wolff, L., et al, Paraplegia Following Intrathecal Cytosine
   Arabinoside.
   Cancer, 43: 83-85, 1979.
15.Young, R.C., et al, Central Nervous System Complications of Non-
   Hodgkin's Lymphoma.
   Amer.J.Med., 66: 435-443, 1979.

19. SUBDURAL HAEMATOMA DUE TO MENINGEAL METASTASIS

J.A.M. Frederiks

Most intracranial metastases are in the cerebrum and the cerebellum. The localization of metastatic malignant disease in the dura mater is very rare (1).Recently we observed a most unusual case of subdural haematoma.Firstly because it recurred,secondly because it originated from metastatic lung carcinoma and thirdly because the haematoma was antemortem the only clinical manifestation of malignant disease of the lung.

These findings prompted me to report this case together with a review of the literature on subdural haematoma due to metastatic malignant disease.In my view our experience has some consequences for the treatment of patients with malignant disease presenting disorders of consciousness or other neurological problems.

Case Report

A 54-year-old man was admitted for the first time with progressive headache,nauseas and diplopia.His gait was unsteady.The past history reveals only a heart attack 3 years before.No trauma.On admission he appeared pale and sick.He had some difficulty in concentrating,but was alert.Normal blood pressure,and no neurological abnormalities.No signs of meningeal irritation.The CSF pressure showed increased pressure of 25 cm of water.The fluid was clear and colourless and c ontained 9 lymphocytes and 12 erythrocytes.The protein was 68,5 mg%,the sugar 3,4 mmol/l.Normal serological tests and immunoelectrophoresis. Repeated lumbar punctures revealed a low pressure,a yellow colour,some erythrocytes.After centrifuge the fluid contained haemoglobin and bilirubin.On extensive examination blood and urine showed normal values except for a slightly increased sedimentation rate.Normal ECG and EEG on admission,but at the time of the third lumbar puncture the EEG showed diffuse slow activity with a maximum left frontotemporal. Normalbrain scintigraphical examination with technetium.On neuro-psychological examination no focal signs were elicited.The patient

showed slight disturbances of consciousness.No abnormalities on x-rays
of skull and thorax.Seldinger angiography of the cerebral vessels
showed slight arteriosclerotic signs of some intracerebral vessels but
but no signs of intracranial process.

The condiotion of the patient worsened.He showed signs of increased
intracranial pressure in the 6th week of admission,including papil-
oedema.No abnormalities on examination of other organ systems.

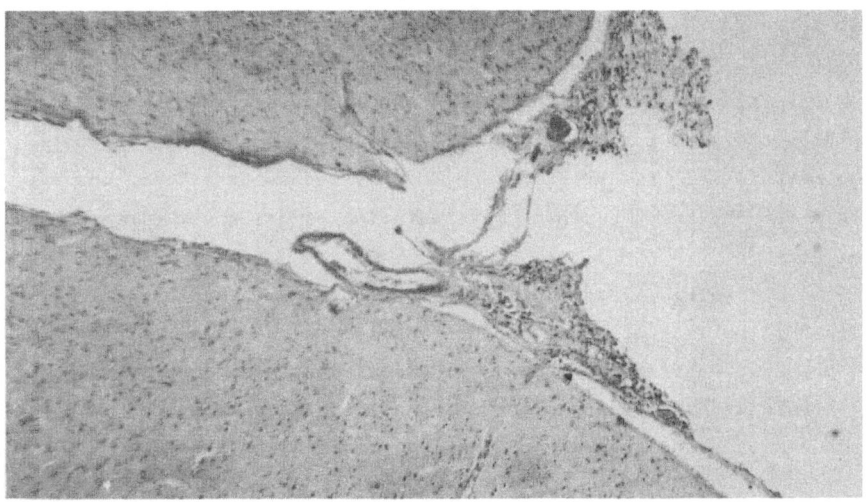

Figure 1

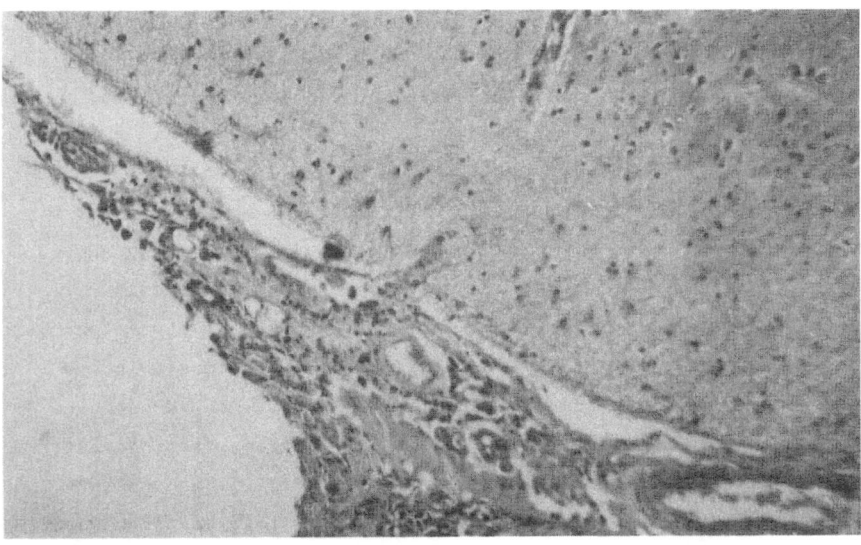

Figure 2

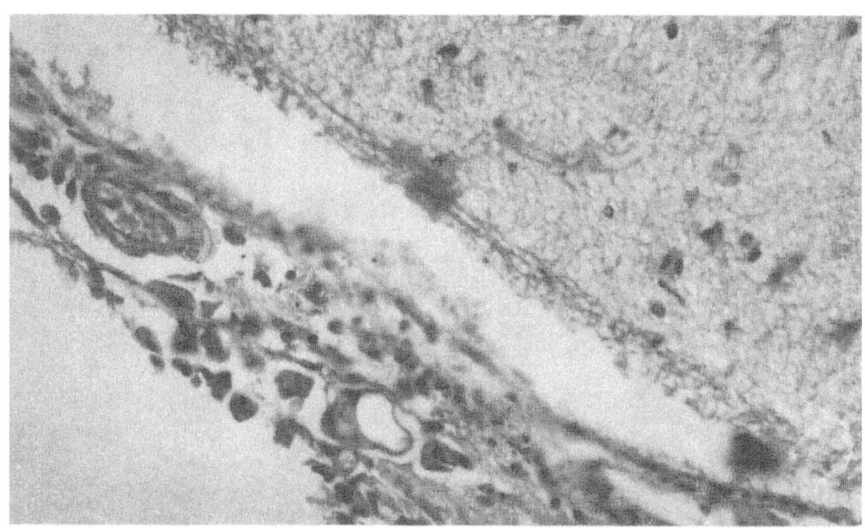

Figure 3

(Figures 1,2 and 3: Sulcus cortex cerebri showing meninges and
malignant cells. x100,x250, and x400 respectively)

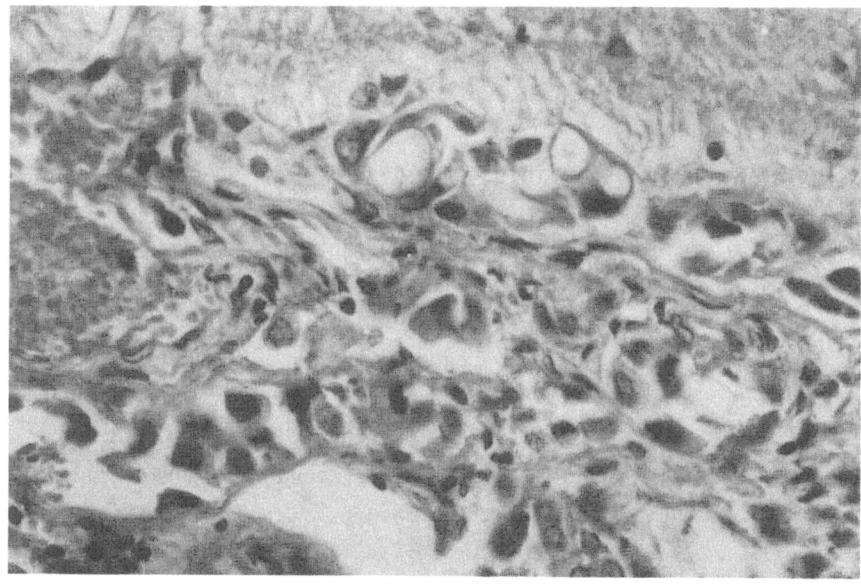

Figure 4

(Microphotograph showing undifferentiated greatcellular metastatic
place in the meninges. x400).

222

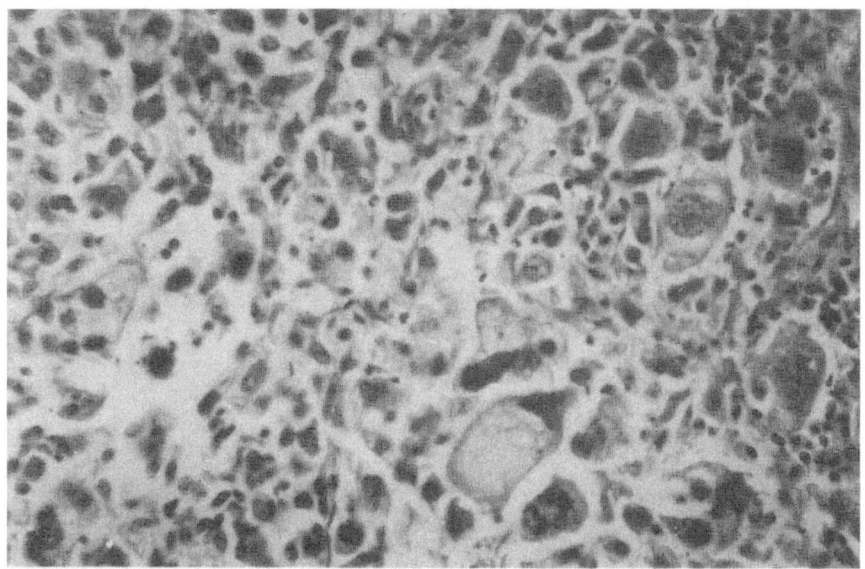

Figure 5

(A microscopic section of the lung tumor:undifferentiated greatcellular carcinoma. x250).

A second angiography of the cerebral vessels showed a thick subdural
haematoma with localization left parietal region.The patient was
operated upon the next day and the haematoma was removed.There was no
membrane.Recovery was complete.But some days following discharge he
again complained of headache and nausea and drowsiness.The headache
was worse in sitting or standing positions,but decreased in horizontal
position of the body.He showed papiloedema,Babinski sign on the right
side and drowsiness.The CSF showed a low pressure of 4 cm of water.
This CSF showed some polymorph cells at the third cell preparation,
suspect of an astrocytoma.Re-examination was necessary into the nature
of a probably underlying disease causing the subdural haematoma
(brain tumor? metastatic tumor?).A pulmonary tumor was not found.Any
other examination failed to reveal a malignant distant disease or
brain disease.But a subdural haematoma was found and operated upon.
During the observation the patient showed a clear syndrome of
orthostatic headache and nausea,presenting a CSF hypotension syndrome.
Repeated extensive examination did not reveal disturbance of other
organ systems.Full examination for occult malignant disease was
negative,but the patient had two recurrences of the subdural haematoma
at the same localization.The patient was operated upon three times.He

died 5 months after the first admission.Except for the last CSF,
examined after the third operation,suspected cells were found.
On postmortem examination was found: 1) A status after craniotomy for
subdural haematoma left parieto-temporal.The dura was adherent to the
skull on several places.The meninges were thickened due to carcinomatosis of the meninges reaching deep into the sulci.No intracerebral
metastases.Xanthogromatous colouring of dura mater and old blood
between dura mater and the leptomeninges. 2) An undifferentiated
greatcellular carcinoma of the lung (right,upper lobè)No metastatic
localizations in other organs of the body.See figures 1-5.
In conclusion :a 54-year-old man was operated upon three times because
of recurrent subdural haematoma.Extensive general somatic and
neurological examination in all the stages of admission failed to
reveal a cause of this recurrent bleeding:no blood disorder,no systematic or local malignant disease was found.On postmortem examination,
however,a carcinoma of the lung was found.There were metastases in the
meninges at the localization of the recurrent subdural haematoma.No
cerebral metastases,and no metastases in other organs of the body.As
to the clinical features it was remarkable to notice orthostatic
headache and vomiting and a CSF hypotension syndrome.The recurrent
subdural haematoma in this patient formed the only clinical manifestation of lung carcinoma.

Discussion

This case leads me to a small discussion about two aspects of subdural
haematoma.Firstly,the problem of recurrent subdural haematoma and
secondly,the problem of subdural haematoma in association with
malignant disease of the meninges.

A) Recurrent subdural haematoma

No knowledge exists of the frequency in which recurrence of subdural
haematoma occurs.We only know the paper of McLaurin and Tutor (2).They
analysed the follow-up facts of ninety cases of acute subdural
haematoma.Of this series 57 died,in 34 of these cases autopsy was
performed and in 9 cases there was a recurrence of the haematoma.All
the 90 cases were operated upon in the first 25 hours following head
injury.There were no cases of malignant disease.

From a clinical point of view one always must differentiate
between postoperative cerebral oedema and recurrence of the haematoma.
This may pose difficult diagnostic dicisions and management.

TABLE

author	age	sexe	side	trauma?	recurrent?	cer.meta.?	operation?	autopsy?	pos.CSF cells?	diagnosis before death	organ	histological diagnosis
Westenhoeffer (1904)	29	F	bil.	-	-	-	-	+	-	at autopsy	stomach	carcinoma
Russell et al. (1934)	64	M	R	-	-	-	+	-	-	at operat.	sinus?	carcinoma
,,	65	F	R	-	-	-	-	+	-	at autopsy	stomach	carcinoma
,,	44	M	bil.	-	-	-	-	+	-	at autopsy	lung	carcinoma
,,	41	M	L	-	-	-	-	+	-	at autopsy	bone	myelosarcoma
Braun (1963)	48	F	bil.	-	-	-	+	+	-	at operat.	stomach	adenocarcinoma
McDonald et al. (1966)	43	M	R	+	-	-	+	+	-	at angiogr.	diffuse	Hodgkin's disease
Pirker et al. (1967)	?	?	R	-	-	-	+	+	-	at angiogr.	pancreas	adenocarcinoma
Kothandaram (1970)	2,5	M	bil.	-	-	-	+	+	-	at angiogr.	dura mater	liposarcoma
Krempien (1970)	56	F	R	-	-	-	-	+	-	at autopsy	mamma	adenocarcinoma
C.S. (1972)	71	M	bil.	-	-	-	-	+	-	at autopsy	pancreas	adenocarcinoma

TABLE (continued)

author	age	sexe	side	trauma?	recurrent?	cer.meta.?	operation?	autopsy?	pos.CSF cells?	diagnosis before death	organ	histological diagnosis
Tzonos et al. (1972)	2,5	F	bil.	+	+	-	+	+	-	at operat.	meninges	sarcoma
Braun et al. (1973)	53	M	L	-	-	-	-	+	-	at autopsy	?	anaplastic carcinoma
Leech et al. (1974)	62	F	bil.	-	-	-	+	+	-	at angiogr.	pancreas	adenocarcinoma

As to the possible causes of recurrency several points must be
mentioned:

1) Failure of the brain to expand after haematoma evacuation (3,4,5).
One sometimes prevents recurrence by applying a subdural drain for
24-48 hours.A craniotomy instead of burr holes is recommended.To check
the expension of the brain,silver clips can be applied to the dura and
the cortex.These and other surgical preventive aspects are discussed
by several authors (4,6).

2) Dehydration (humoral factors) may give rise to collapse and in this
way to recurrence of the haematoma (7).

3) Recurrence of the haematoma also may occur in the presence of
infections or invasion of the meninges by leucemic cells (8).

4) Bleeding diathesis (for instance anticoagulant therapy,blood
disease).

5) Metastases to the meninges (the case presented in this paper).

B) Subdural haematoma from meningeal metastatic malignant disease

Meningeal metastases of malignant disease are rare (9).The occurrence
of subdural haematoma in those cases is very rare (1).

Meyer and Reah (10) presented 20 cases of diffuse dural metastases of
which 9 cases had also a "pac hymeningitis haemorrhagica interna"
(4 cases out of these nine have already been described by Russell and
Cairns (11)).In recent years 14 cases have been described more or
less comprehensively.The Table presented in this paper summarizes the
findings of cases of subdural haematoma due to meningeal metastases
of malignant disease.

Only in one of these 14 cases the subdural haematoma was recurrent;
seven were bilateral.

Several arguments as to the pathogenesis have been elecited by
several authors:

1) Obstruction of dural vessels by tumor cells (1,11) is the most
generally accepted explanation.Other presented explanations in
rare cases have been:

2) Vascular and fibrous proliferation associated with intravascular
growth (tumor-induced angiodesmoplasia).The subdural haematoma results
from bleeding into this highly vascular abnormal areolar layer of
the dura (12).

3) An uncommon case has been described about a mucine-producing
adenocarcinoma giving rise to subdural effusion of fluid and blood
(13).

4) Another uncommon case has been described with bleeding diathesis associated with meningeal metastases of an adenocarcinoma from the pancreas (12).

To sum up one can state that in each case suspected of subdural haematoma in a patient with malignant disease,a lumbar puncture is indicated with careful examination of the CSF cells and with a careful registration of the CSF pressure.

Subdural haematoma with meningeal metastases f om malignant disease is rare,but one should always think of this possibility if a patient with malignant disease becomes drowsy and presents ortho-static symptoms of headache and nausea (CSF hypotension syndrome).

In uncommon presentation of a subdural haematoma one should consider the desirability to make a craniotomy instead of burr holes (6,14).In the presence of suspicion of malignant disease, pathological examination of a biopsy of the haematoma-membrane and haematoma-material is a necessity.This in association with cytology of the CSF cells may be of value in treating these diagnostic and therapeutic difficult to manage cases of subdural haematoma.

REFERENCES

1. Braun EM,LJ Burger and HA Schlang:Subdural hematoma from meta-static malignant disease.Cancer (Philad.) 32:1370-1373,1973

2. McLaurin RL,FT Tutor:Acute subdural haematoma.Review of ninety cases.J.Neurosurg.18:61-67,1961

3. Trotter W:Chronic subdural haemorrhage of traumatic origin and its relation to pachymeningitis haemorrhagica interna.Brit.J.Surg. 2:271-291,1914

4. Robinson RG:The treatment of subacute and chronic subdural haematomas.Brit.med.J.1:21-22,1955

5. Hancock DO:Cerebral collapse associated with chronic subdural haematoma in adults.Lancet 1:633-634,1965

6. Van der Werf AJM:Surgical management of acute subdural hematomas. Clin.Neurol.Neurosurg. 78:161-170,1975

7. Chavany JA,B Pertuiset,B Weil and D.Hagenmuller:Les troubles humoraux observés aux cóurs de l'évolution d'un hématome sous-dural spontané et récidivant.Mschr.Psychiatr.Neurol.

12 8:315-326,1954

8. De Reuck J,H Roels and H vander Eecken:Complications of the chronic subdural haematoma.Clin.Neurol.Neurosurg.79:203-210,1976

9. Hengefeld JW,JWA Sweh,PM Bakker and LJ Endtz:Carcinomatose van de hersenvliezen.Ned.T.Geneesk.122:1875-1880.1978

10. Meyer PC and TG Reah:Secondary neoplasms of the central nervous system and meninges.Brit.J.Cancer 7:438-448,1953

11. Russell DS and H Cairns:Subdural false membrane or haematoma (pachymeningitis interna haemorrhagica) in carcinomatosis and sarcomatosis of the dura mater.Brain 57:32-48,1934

12. Leech RW,FT Welch and GA Ojemann:Subdural hematoma secondary to metastatic dural carcinomatosis.Case report.J.Neurosurg.14: 610-613,19 74

13. CR:Case 12-1972 Massachusetts general hospital.New Engl.J.med.186: 650-656,1972

14. Biemond A:Hersenziekten.Haarlem,De Erven F.Bohn,1961

15. Westenhoeffer M:Pachymeningitis carcinomatosa haemorrhagica interna productiva mit Colibacillosis agonalis.Virchows Archiff 1 75:364-3 79,1904

16. Braun W:Ein subdurales Hämatom als Folge einer metastatischen Karzinomatose der harten Hirnhaut.Zbl.Neurochir.23:210-215,1963

1 7. McDonald JV and R Burton:Subdural effusion in Hodgkin's disease. Arch.Neurol.15:649-652,1966

18. Pirker E and HE Diemath:Besonderkeiten bei Subduralhämatomen. Röntgenfortschritte 106:231-235,1967

19. Kothandaram P:Dural liposarcoma associated with subdural hematoma. Case report.J.Neurosurg.33: 85-87,1970

20. Krempien B:Durahygrom bei Carcinose der harten Hirnhaut.Zentralbl. Allg.Pathol.113:409-414,19 70

21. Tzonos T an d B Kraus:Subduraler Erguss als Folge eines diffusen Leptomeningealsarkoms.Neurochir.(Stuttgart) 6:227-231,1972

20. CLINICAL ASPECTS OF MENINGEAL CARCINOMATOSIS

J.W.A. Swen, J.W. Hengefeld, L.J. Endtz

Although carcinomatous meningitis is a good descriptive
term, the lesion is purely neoplastic and signs of meningitis are not always present. It therefore seems more appropriate to speak of meningeal carcinomatosis. This affection
is a diffuse or widespread multifocal seeding of the leptomeninges of the brain and spinal cord by a metastatic tumour. Eberth (1) gave the first description of a patient
with this clinical picture. Recent reports indicate that
this complication of systemic cancer is a still increasing
problem (2,3). Because the blood-brain barrier prevents
many anti-neoplastic drugs from reaching the central nervous system, it is extremely difficult to treat metastasis
beyond this barrier.

According to Hildebrand et al. (4), this meningeal spread
of tumour cells is seen in leucaemic processes and less
frequently in carcinoma of the lung, breast, and digestive
tract, and malignant lymphomas. Some authors (2) include
cases with neurological symptoms referable to tumour seeding of the meninges or neural structures in contact with
the meninges or both, whereas others (5-7) exclude cases
with parenchymatous lesions. In a prospective autopsy investigation of 1,096 cases, Chason (8) found 200 with central nervous system metastases, and focal and/or diffuse
involvement of the leptomeninges in 116 (58%). In 100 cases
the affected area was limited to the region overlying parenchymatous metastases. Diffuse carcinomatosis was found
in 16 cases (8%). Only one had no parenchymatous lesions.

The mechanisms mainly responsible for the syndrome of meningeal carcinomatosis are: direct invasion of the spinal or
cranial nerves from the subarachnoïd space; invasion of the
cerebral or spinal cord parenchyme from the Virchow-Robin
spaces; and obstruction of CSF pathways.

Clinical features of the present series

Our series comprises 16 patients (3 women and 13 men) with
a solid tumour who developed meningeal carcinomatosis between January, 1976 and January, 1979. Their ages ranged
between 27 and 76 years, with a mean age of 57 years. At
the time of diagnosis the primary tumour was not known in 9
cases (56%). In the other 7 cases (44%) a primary tumour
had been found 4 to 84 months earlier.

TABLE I   The main signs and symptoms in 16 patients with
          meningeal carcinomatosis.

Signs and symptoms	Number of patients	Per-cen-tage
cranial nerve lesions	9	56
headache	8	50
radiculopathy	7	43
disturbance of consciousness	6	37
micturition disorders	6	37
neck stiffness	4	25
paraplegia	4	25
disturbance of behaviour	3	19
unilateral paresis	3	19
nausea, vomiting	2	12
polyneuropathy	1	6

The most important complaints (table I) at admission were
functional deficiency due to a cranial nerve disorder (56%),
headache (50%), or pain extending to one or both legs (43%).
Three patients developed a cranial nerve lesion as the
disease progressed. During the period of observation we
saw a functional deficiency of various cranial nerves
(table 2).

TABLE 2 Cranial   nerve lesions   in the present series

Cranial nerve	Number of patients
olfactory	1
optic	2
oculomotor	2
abducens	4
facial	2
cochleovestibular	4
hypoglossal	2

Three patients had more than one cranial nerve lesion. The high frequency of lesions of the optic and cochleovestibular nerve is stressed in the literature (9-11). Disorders of micturition (37%) disturbance of consciousness (37%), para-plegia (25%), and neck stiffness (25%), were less frequent. On admission, all patients were conscious; 6 were somnolent or soporous. In all patients with a micturition disorder, compression of the caudal nerves was responsible for the neurogenic bladder dysfunction. Nausea and vomiting (12%), psychiatric syndromes (19%), unilateral paresis (19%), and polyneuropathy were relatively infrequent. One patient pre-sented with delirium tremens and was initially transferred to a psychiatric hospital. Two other patients seemed to be disoriented. Of the patients with unilateral paresis (19%), none showed parenchymatous metastases at autopsy. EEG and isotope scans were negative in these latter cases.

Additional investigations

As Prentice a.o. (12, 13) pointed out as early as 1973, caudal myelography can be of great value in establishing the
diagnosis. This is illustrated by one of our patients, in
whom caudal myelography (figure 1) showed multiple nodular
filling defects.

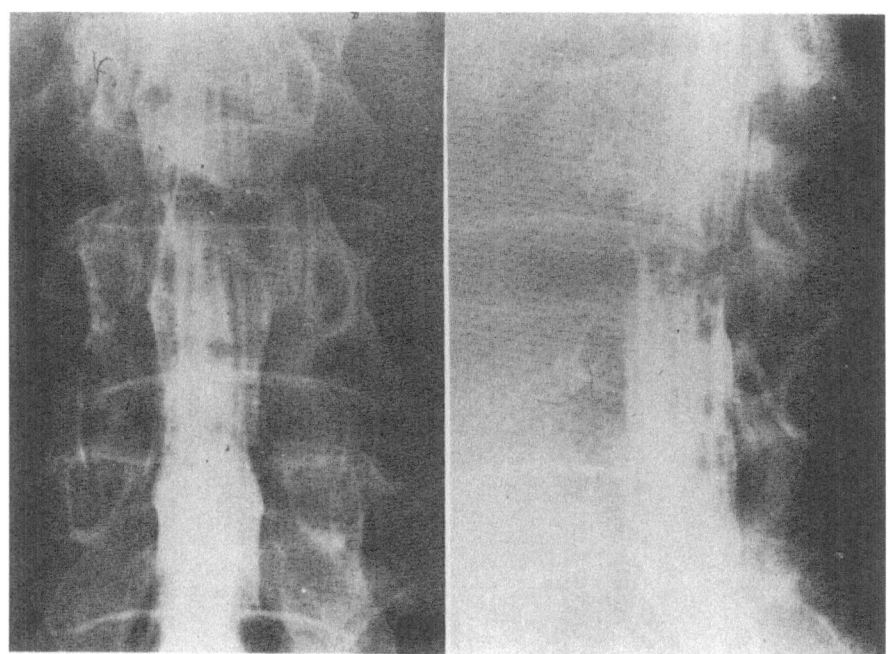

Figure 1. Caudal myelography showing multiple nodular
filling defects at the level of L III.

234

At autopsy, multiple small tumours were found in and around the caudal nerves (figure 2).

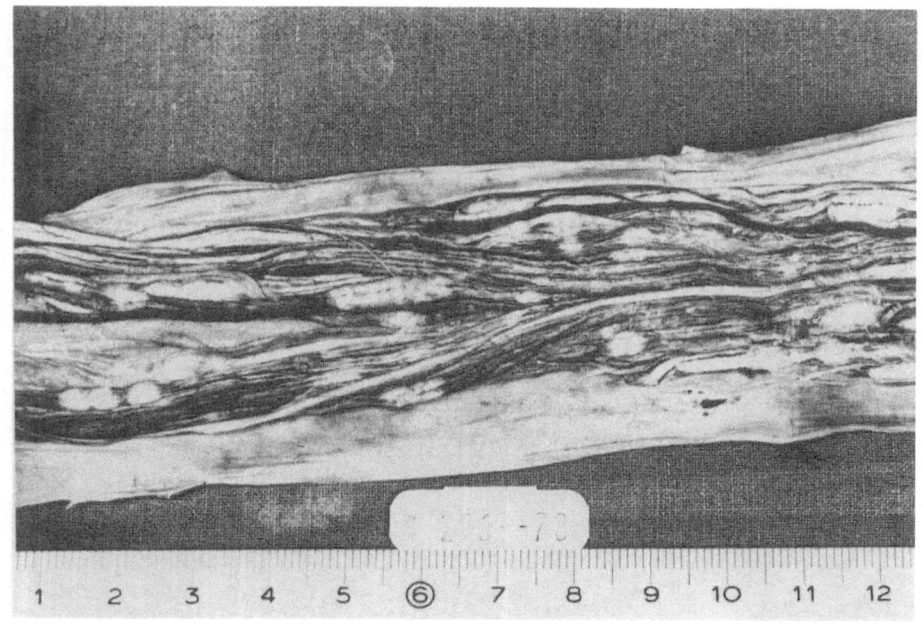

Figure 2: Multiple small tumours in the cauda equina.

Histologically, these tumours showed invasion of nerves in some cases (figure 3), whereas in others invasion had not occured.

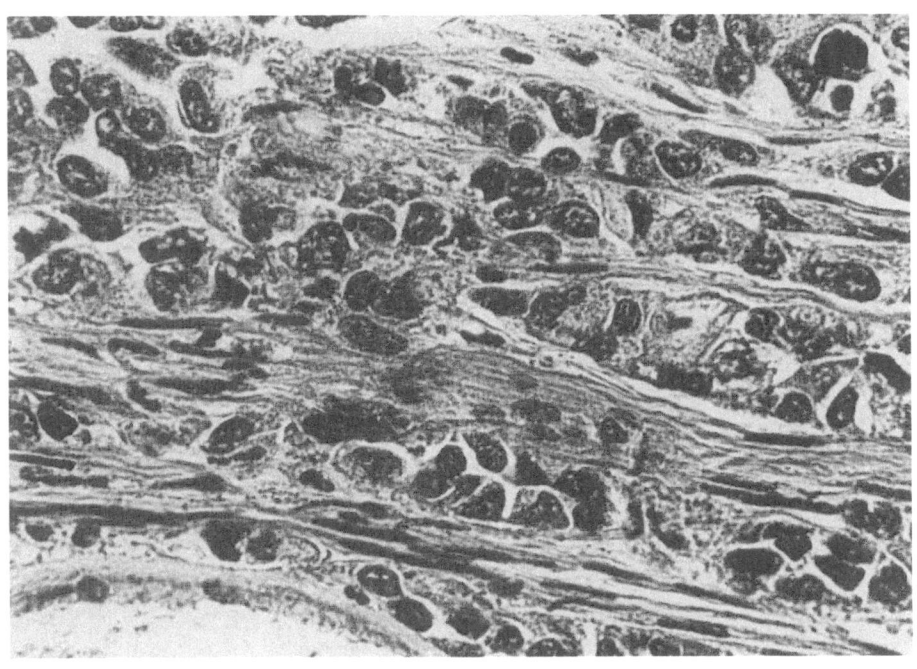

Figure 3: Histologically distinct invasion of caudal roots
by tumour cells.

In four cases myelography did not provide useful   information about pathological changes.
Electromyography was performed in 7 cases with radicular
symptoms. Six patients showed fibrillation. The other patient died 4 days after admission, which might explain this
negative result. Skull X-rays were made in 5 cases and
showed small osteolytic abnormalities in one of them. On
routine EEG, three out of 16 patients clearly showed focal
disturbances. In one case a focus with slow wave activity
was found that could have been due to a metastasis but an
isotope scan was normal and no clinical signs of a cerebral
hemisphere lesion were present. This patient proved to have
carcinomatosis of the caudal leptomeninges. The second of
these patients suffered from a spontaneous subdural haematoma. In this case histology revealed extensive outgrowth

of tumour cells in the surrounding leptomeninges. In the
third patient the presence of intracerebral metastasis in
the right occipital lobe was confirmed by a CAT scan. She
was admitted with a radicular syndrome and later developed
a caudal syndrome with a normal myelograph. After approximately 170 days of treatment, she developed symptoms of a cerebral hemisphere lesion. At autopsy, meningeal carcinomatosis of the cerebral and caudal leptomeninges was found.

Cerebrospinal fluid examination
In two cases a lumber puncture was not performed. The following data concern the other 14 cases (table 3).

TABLE 3   Findings in the cerebrospinal fluid in the
present series.

		Number of patients	percentage
opening pressure (N=14)	elevated in	5	36
leucocytes (N=14)	increased in (range 4-480/mm^3)	13	93
cytology (N=11)	positive in	11	100
protein (N=14)	increased in (range 0.73-7.3 g/l)	14	100
glucose (N=8)	decreased in	6	75

The pressure was initially elevated in 5 cases, normal in 8,
and not known in one. The leucocyte number varied from 4 to
480 per mm^3. In 3 cases cytological examination was omitted.
In all other cases the sedimentation preparation made according to Sayk (16, 17) showed malignant cells (14, 15). In
two cases the sedimentation study had to be repeated twice
before positive results were obtained. The protein content
was elevated in all cases. The CSF glucose level was not

determined in 6 cases; in 2 cases it was normal and in 6 out
of 8 cases was lower than 2/3 of the blood level (18).
Differential diagnostic problems may arise in patients with
a mycotic or bacterial infection of the leptomeninges (19),
especially tuberculosis. In our series 2 patients were primarily treated for a possible tuberculous meningitis.

Course

The course was invariably fatal in our series. The duration
varied from 1 to 192 days. The patients can be divided into two
groups: one treated (N=7) and the other untreated (N=9). Because the therapeutic approach was changed during the period
under consideration, no conclusions can be drawn about the
effect on the course, but we have the impression that doing
nothing is the worst of all. The therapy applied seemed to
be at least a palliative kind of treatment for unbearable
pain. What we actually saw after treatment was a normaliza-
tion of the increased CSF pressure and a decrease in the
number of tumour cells. The elevated protein level tended
to normalize, as did the decreased glucose level. With respect to the patients' complaints: the headache and stiffness
of the neck decreased and the radicular pain strongly diminished during treatment.

Pathology

Autopsy was not performed in 3 cases, in two of which the
primary tumour had already been demonstrated. In these 3 cases the diagnosis had been based on the clinical and cytological findings. In the other cases the localization of the
tumour in the leptomeninges was verified by the autopsy
findings. The primary tumour was identified in all but 2
cases (table 4).

TABLE 4   Primary tumour in 16 patients with meningeal carcinomatosis

Type	Site	Number of patients
Adenocarcinoma	lung	3
	prostate	2
	breast	1
Undifferentiated Carcinoma	lung	5
	breast	1
Squamous cell carcinoma	ethmoid sinus	1
Hypernephroma	kidney	1
Unknown origin		2

Six cases concerned adenocarcinomas: 3 of the lungs, 2 of the prostate, and one of the breast; 5 patients showed an undifferentiated lung carcinoma and one an undifferentiated breast tumour. One case concerned a squamous cell carcinoma derived from an ethmoid sinus and another a hypernephroma originating from a kidney. In 2 cases the primary tumour remained unknown, although adenocarcinoma cells were found in the CSF.

At autopsy, 2 patients (15%) showed no signs of metastasis beyond the regional lymph nodes. In all of the other cases multiple metastases were found outside the CNS. Three cases (30%) had intracerebral parenchymatous lesions; 2 of these cases have already been discussed, and in the last no clini-cal signs of an intracerebral lesion were found retrospec-tively.

The histopathogenesis has been discussed elsewhere (20).

Conclusions
The clinical picture of meningeal carcinomatosis is characterized by an insidious onset and a progressive course un-
till death. The clinical manifestations can be divided into
4 categories: 1. meningeal irritation and neck rigidity, 2.
irritation or functional deficit of the cranial or spinal
nerves, particularly of the cauda equina; 3. psychiatric
syndromes, probably as a result of a rise of intracranial
pressure, and 4. abnormalities of the cerebral spinal fluid.

Generally, the patient had symptoms of structural disease
involving the neuraxis at more than one place. Cytological
examination of the cerebral spinal fluid, as well as a specific history and a characteristic clinical picture, are
essential for the diagnosis. Lumbar puncture has to be repeated in some cases before the diagnosis can be established.
A positive cytological picture alone does not exclude the
possibility of an intracerebral or primary meningeal tumour
(17, 21). Aspecific alterations may also be found, for instance a rise of the CSF pressure, leucocytosis, an elevated
protein level, or a decreased glucose level.
Meningeal carcinomatosis is frequently the first manifestation of metastasis of a primary solid tumour, as in our series (56%), and may be the only metastatic process beyond
the regional lymph nodes (15%). Meningeal carcinomatosis
can also be present in patients with a parenchymatous lesion.
In that case the pathogenesis is possibly different but the
clinical picture is the same. It seems possible that as time
goes on metastatic invasion occurs from the perivascular
spaces into the parenchyme.
Finally, our limited experience with intrathecal therapy
indicates that it is better to attempt treatment than to
do nothing, and that one should never forget that since one
or more tumours are present elsewhere in the body as well,
the therapy for meningeal carcinomatosis must be integrated
into some form of systemic therapy.

240

REFERENCES

1. Eberth, CJ, Zur Entwickelung des Epithelioms der Pia und der Lunge. Virchow's Arch path Anat und Physiologie. 49 : 51-63, 1870.

2. Olsen, ME, NL Chernik and JB Posner, Infiltration of the Leptomeninges by Systemic Cancer. Arch Neurol 30 : 122-137, 1974.

3. Little, JR, AJD Dale and H Okazaki, Meningeal Carcinomatosis. Arch Neurol 30 : 138-143, 1974.

4. Hildebrand, J and L Debusscher, Meningeal Carcinomatosis, In: Recent advances in Cancer Treatment. Tagnon, HJ (ed.), New York, Raven, 241-253, 1977.

5. Chobaut, JC, B Brichet, C Petit, JM Friot and M Wayoff, Meningite carcinomateuse métastatique d'origine ORL. Oto -Neuro-Opht 50 : 151-159, 1978.

6. Buge, A, D Fohanno and F Gray, L'hypertension intracrânienne des méningites carcinomateuses. Ann Med interne 128 : 2, 143-149, 1977.

7. Fischer-Williams, M, FD Bosanquet and PM Daniel, Carcinomatosis of the meninges. Brain 78 : 42-58, 1955.

8. Chason, JL, FB Walker and JW Landers. Metastatic carcinoma in the central nervous system and dorsal root ganglia. Cancer (Philad.) 16 : 781-786, 1963.

9 Altrocchi, PH and PB Eckman, Meningeal carcinomatosis and blindness. J Neurol Neurosurg Psychiat 36 : 206-210, 1973.

10. Appen RE, G de Venecia, JH Selliken and LT Giles, Meningeal carcinomatosis with blindness. Amer J Ophtal 86 : 661-665, 1978.

11. Alberts, MC and CF Terrence, Hearing loss in carcinomatous meningitis. J Laryngol Otol 92 : 233-241, 1978.

12. Prentice, WB, SA Kieffer, LHA Gold and RGB Bjornson, Myelographic characteristics of metastasis to the spinal cord and cauda equina, Amer J Roentgenol 118 : 682-689, 1973.

13. Bobroff, LM and NE Leeds, Minimal terminal irregularities of the distal subarachnoid space as a sign of epidural seeding. Amer J Roentgenol 118: 601-604, 1973.

14. Balhuizen, JC, GThAM Bots, A Schaberg and FT Bosman,

Value of cerebrospinal fluid cytology for the diagnosis of malignancies in the central nervous system . J Neurosurg 48 : 747-753, 1978.

15. Glass, JP, M Melamed, ML Chernik and JB Posner, Malignant cells in cerebrospinal fluid. Neurology 29 : 1369-1375, 1979.

16. Sayk, J, Ergebnisse neuer liquor cytologischer Untersuchungen mit dem Sedimentierkammer Verfahren. Artz Wchnschr 9 : 1042-1046, 1954.

17. Den Hartog Jager, WA, Cytopathology of the cerebrospinal fluid examined with the sedimentation technique after Sayk. J Neurol Sci 9 : 155-177, 1969.

18. De Vita, VT and GP Canellos, Hypoglycorrhagia in meningeal carcinomatosis. Cancer (Philad.) 19 : 691-694,1966.

19. Morganroth, J, A Deisseroth, S Winokur and P Schein, Differentiation of carcinomatous and bacterial meningitis. Neurology 22 : 1240-1242, 1972.

20. Hengefeld, JW, JWA Swen, PM Bakker and LJ Endtz, Carcinomatose van de hersenvliezen. Ned T Geneesk 122 : 1875 -1880, 1978.

21. Daum S and JF Foncin, Les tumeurs diffuses des leptoméninges. Rev Neurol 108 : 597-612, 1963.

21. TREATMENT OF MENINGEAL LEUCAEMIA, MENINGEAL LYMPHOMA AND CARCINOMATOSIS

R. Somers, Z.D. Goedhart, B.W. Ongerboer de Visser

Introduction

Before the introduction of the central nervous system (CNS) prophylaxis in acute lymphoblastic leucaemia (ALL) in childhood the incidence of meningeal leucaemia was about 50%. Now it is only 10%, but
extension to the meninges might become more frequent in the near future, due to a better patient survival. Simultaneous the incidence
of meningeal metastases from certain types of malignant lymphoma, such
as mediastinal T-cell lymphoma in children and young adults and in
hystiocytic lymphoma stage IV, is increasing. Breast cancer, lung cancer and melanoma are the solid tumors which may cause meningeal involvement. The symptoms have been described in the previous paper by
Swen. It is the purpose of our paper to discuss the treatment of meningeal metastases and specially the role of the ventriculostomy system (V.S.) of Ommaya (O.S.). Finally the pharmacology and toxicity of
MTX will be considered.

II. The Ommaya System: surgical aspects and clinical use

Drugs can be directly administered to the cerebrospinal fluid (CSF)
via the lumbar or ventricular route. In this connection MTX is the
drug with which there is the most experience. Both routes have their
advantages and disadvantages.

Advantages of the lumbar route:
1. the cytological CSF examination is usually more reliable
2. the infection rate is almost zero per cent.
Disadvantages of the lumbar route:
1. because the intracranial pressure (ICP) may be increased in meningeal extension of malignancies or the clinical picture resembles
   that of raised ICP, it is not possible to differentiate between

provocation or aggravation of a cerebellar herniation

2. in a concommitent herniation, which compromises the CSF pathways, lumbar puncture (L.P.) gives no accurate information about the ICP. Furthermore the obtained CSF levels of MTX are not representative

3. lumbar injection of MTX produces insufficient and inconstant intra-cranial MTX levels (Shapiro 1975)

4. treatment via the lumbar route may be very inconvenient for the pa-tient due to the necessity for repeated punctures and painfull in-jections.

The disadvantages of the ventricular route are:

1. counting of the pathological cells in the CSF is less reliable

2. the very substantial cerebral damage of repetitive transcerebral punctures

3. the necessity of an operatively created entry (except in small in-fants with an open fontanelle).

After a consideration of the advantages and disadvantages of each route we feel that the ventricular route is the better method. However a burr-hole permits a blunt ventricular puncture for only two weeks after which the very dangerous sharp ventricular needles are necessary to tap the ventricular fluid. The V.S. eliminates this pro-blem or will as having other advantages:

1. after one blunt ventricular puncture there is a stable system and therefore also the most minimal cerebral damage

2. puncturing of the reservoir is possible for 100 times over years (Goedhart 1978)

3. the ICP measurements are objective

4. the MTX levels are more representative

5. the radio-isotope ventriculography is more reliable

6. the route of treatment is convenient for the patient and the phy-sician.

The only real problem with the type of V.S. we use is the infection rate, which can be 15% or higher. A suggestion to decrease infection will be given later in this chapter.

Figure 1 shows the O.S. we use in cross-section. This is one of the four types now available (Ommaya 1963). Implantation of this system

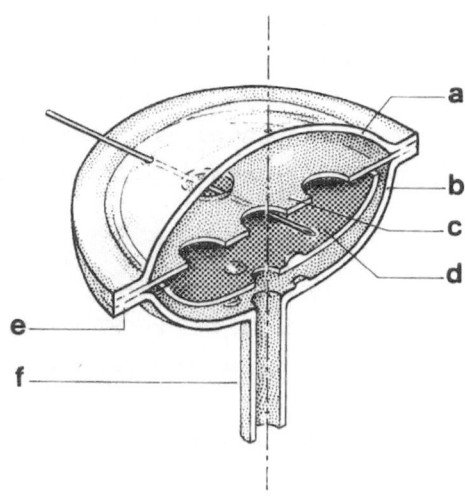

Fig. 1. Cross-section of a burr-hole reservoir with an inner diameter of 1,5 cm. a.is the self-seeling dome, b.the dome on the dural side, c.the perforable mid-membrane, d.a floating hard shell which prevents perforating of b, e.a wing of which the reservoir rests on the margins of the burr-hole, f.the reservoir part of the ventricular catheter.

is contraindicated when the thrombotest is lower than 40%, the granulocytes are less than 1000/cu mm or the platelets lower than 80.000/cu mm.

Figure 2 shows the type of incision we use for the different layers of the scalp. The curved skin incision gives the additional comfort of painless puncturing of the reservoir for at least two weeks. Figure 3 shows the place where the system is usually implanted and the direction of the insertion of the ventricular drain. In these patients we puncture only the lateral ventricle and not the third one, because sooner or later the risk of cerebral bleeding can be elevated (Bleyer 1978; Goedhart 1978). If a frontal burr-hole on the right side is contraindicated, e.g. in case of local scalp metastases, a parietal burr-hole on the right side is made.

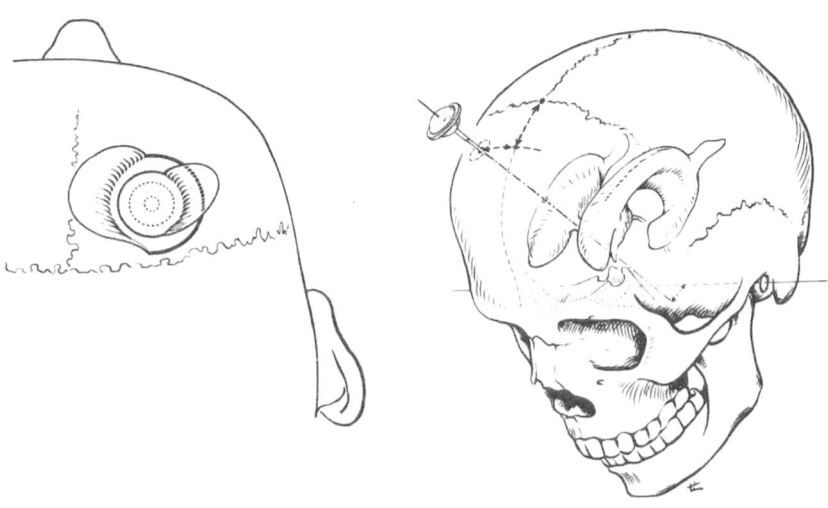

fig. 2   fig. 3

Fig. 2. Precoronal parasagittal burr-hole situated on a line between the two ends of the incision in the skin. The incision in the perios-teum is curved in the opposite direction.

Fig. 3. This three-dimensional drawing shows the parameters applied for the positioning of the drain tip of the OS in the 3rd ventricle.

Puncturing of the reservoir is only performed under sterile conditions, with a 25 G needle and fluid should first be aspirated from the reser-voir to avoid contamination by skin plugs and this sample discharged. The second sample is for bacteriological analysis. After aspiration of the second sample the reservoir must be compressed to refill it with a more representative sample of ventricular fluid. Compressing

of the reservoir is always allowed, because direct postoperational
it is complete stable. The third sample can be used for cytological
and chemical analysis. During the procedure the ICP is measured. After this the MTX is injected and the reservoir compressed again to
spread the injected materials through the ventricles. This procedure
is repeated every time the reservoir is punctured. Bacteriological
analysis is done twice weekly.

In case of contamination of the O.S. the pathogenic micro-organism
is nearly always staphylococcus epidermidis, which grows very slowly
in vitro and vivo. It is therefore advisable to start the above mentioned procedure 24 hours after the implantation of the O.S. Patients
with meningeal malignancies have probably a higher incidence of contamination of the O.S. and therefore we shall start a kind of pre-
treatment with high dose of cefradine (v.d. Waay 1979). When the presence of ventriculitis caused by staphylococcus epidermidis is suspected both intrathecal and systemical treatment with Penicillin G
is commenced whilst awaiting the definite cultures. The only indication for removal of a V.S. in these patients is sepsis.

III. Treatment

There are a number of factors which influence treatment (table 1):
The native and the stage of the primary disease are important. In
metastatic lung cancer and melanoma the rapid progression of the disease itself might prevent treatment of the meningeal extension. In
our experience the presence of solid cerebral metastases seems a con-
traindication to treatment, because of the poor prognosis of these
patients. C.T. scanning is here valuable because of the ease with
which solid metastases can be detected (distinction should be drawn
between publications with and without the above mentioned investigation). Isotope ventriculography with 99m Te-HSA can be a useful in-
dicator of the grade of impairment of the CSF pathways and compression of the ventricles, indicating the sequence of the treatment
(McCullough 1969; Larson 1973).

The most experience in the treatment of meningeal leucaemia, lymphoma
and carcinomatosis has been derived from the treatment of ALL-mening-
geal metastases (Pochedly 1977). From a review of the literature certain guidelines may be formulated. By intrathecal administration of
drugs the CSF can be cleared of leucemic cells with disappearance of

Factors influencing prognosis and treatment decision of meningeal carcinomatosis.

1. Type of tumour.
2. Presence of other tumour localizations outside C.N.S.
3. Presence of other tumour localizations inside C.N.S.
4. Extension of the meningeal carcinomatosis
   - pressure symptoms
   - ventricle compression
   - ventriculographic abnormalities
5. Performance status.
6. Prior chemotherapy or radiotherapy.

Table 1.

symptoms in 90% of the cases. After the remission is reached maintenance treatment is necessary. This can be given by maintenance intrathecal chemotherapy or by consolidation radiotherapy to skull and spine. The radiotherapy dose (2400 - 3000 rad) to the skull is usually higher compared with that given to the spine (1000 - 1500 rad), because the severe myelosuppression, regular accompanying a high dose to the vertebrae, might hamper systematic chemotherapy. It is possible that alternating administration of two drugs, e.g. MTX and cytosine-arabinoside, might give better results but this has get to be confirmed. The role of the high intravenous dose of MTX in the treatment of meningeal leucaemia is not fully settled although therapeutic levels of MTX may be reached, they remain only for a limited period.

The treatment of meningeal involvement in breast cancer with few or no metastases elsewhere is worthwhile with a remission rate of 60%. In lymphomas treatment will also depend on the prior history of the systemic disease. In favourable circumstances the remission rate is 80%. An attractive approach is to start with radiotherapy on the presenting lesion followed by intrathecal administration of MTX (Jap 1979; Shapiro 1977). In cases in which C.T. scanning of the brain is normal and isotope ventriculography shows no gross impairment of the CSF circulation intraventricular administration of drugs can be the first step, followed by radiotherapy to residual lesions if a complete remission is not obtained.

IV. Pharmacokinetics of MTX

When MTX is administered by rapid intravenous injection of normal dose (mg) effective levels of 10^3 nanomol = 10^6 mol in the CSF are not

248

reached (Shapiro 1975). High intravenous dose (1 gram) as used in the treatment of osteosarcoma, produce levels above 10^3 nanomol in the CSF. However they are of short duration and after 24 hours fall below the minimal effective level. Figure 4 shows the MTX levels in the CSF in a group of children treated with i.v. MTX for CNS prophylaxis in leucaemia.

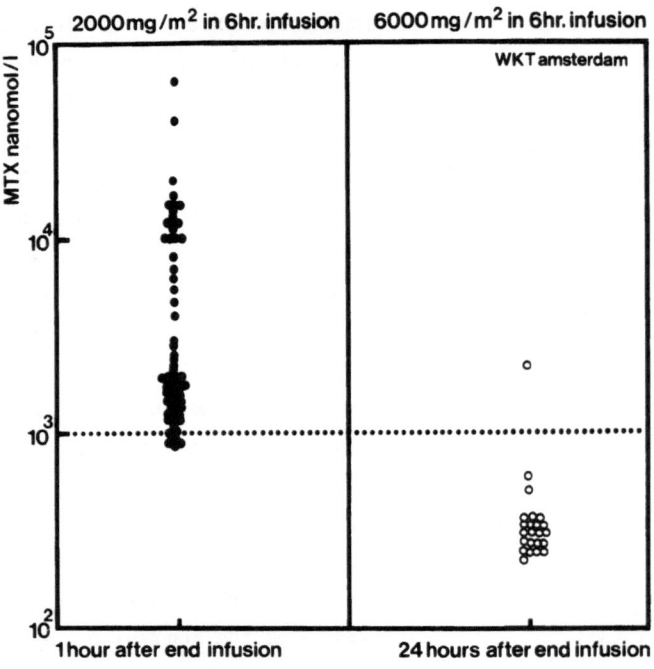

Fig. 4. MTX levels in CSF obtained by lumbar punction 1 hour after the end of 6 hour infusion of 2 g/m2 (left) and 24 hour after the end of 6 hour infusion of 6 g/m2 (right) in children with ALL.

For effective MTX levels of longer duration in the different CSF compartments intraventricular administration is superior to administration via lumbar puncture (Shapiro 1975).

However, after intraventricular administration the duration of the effective levels can differ considerably even in the same patient. After dose of 5 to 10 mg the levels after 24 hours are in the range of 10^5 - 10^6 nanomol/l. and drop below 10^3 nanomol/l. after 48 to 72 hours (figure 5) if the CSF circulation is normal as determined by isotope ventriculography and clearance from the right ventricle (figure 6, patient C). This pattern is changed when there is an abnormal CSF circulation as shown in figure 7. In this patient with meningeal extension of malignant lymphoma and diabetes insipidus the MTX levels remain above 10^4 nanomol/l. 96 and 144 hours after administration. Isotope ventriculography in this patient was abnormal showing a delayed clearance of the isotope (figure 6 ; patient B, before (B) and after treatment (B^1)). Figure 8 shows an improving clearance of the drug in a patient with breast cancer, which parallels an improvement of the neurological symptoms. Figure 9 shows the opposite in a patient with progressive neurological symptoms during treatment: she had also solid metastases deep in the brain beside the third ventricle.

V. Toxicity of intrathecal administration.

Treatment and prophylaxis of meningeal metastases can be complicated by acute and chronic toxicity reactions (table 2) (Pochedly 1977). Several factors (table 3) have been incriminated such as: solvents used for preparation of drugs; solvents in which the drugs are administered; delayed clearance of the drugs caused by the obstructed CSF circulation; kind of drugs administered. Multiple factors might contribute in each case. Using Elliots B solution as a solvent to administer the drug reduces the incidence of toxicity reactions but does not abolish them. Although most acute toxicities are described with the use of MTX, cases have also been noticed in which Ara-C was used. The role of different factors causing the more chronic toxicity reaction as indicated in table 2 has been extensively studied. It seems that the sequence: radiotherapy - intrathecal chemotherapy is important in the pathogenesis of encephalopathy. This especially holds for radiotherapeutic doses aboe 2400 rad. The total dose of drugs administered systematically and intrathecally might also be of importance.

250

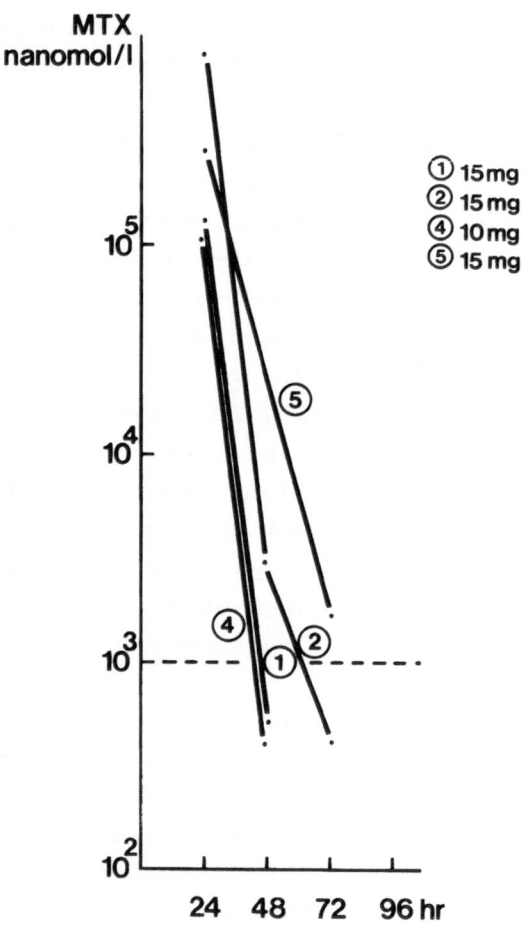

Fig. 5. MTX levels in CSF obtained by Ommaya reservoir puncture in patient C. with ALL meningeal leucaemia. The disappearance of 29 hr Tc+HSA is shown in fig. 6 (patient C).

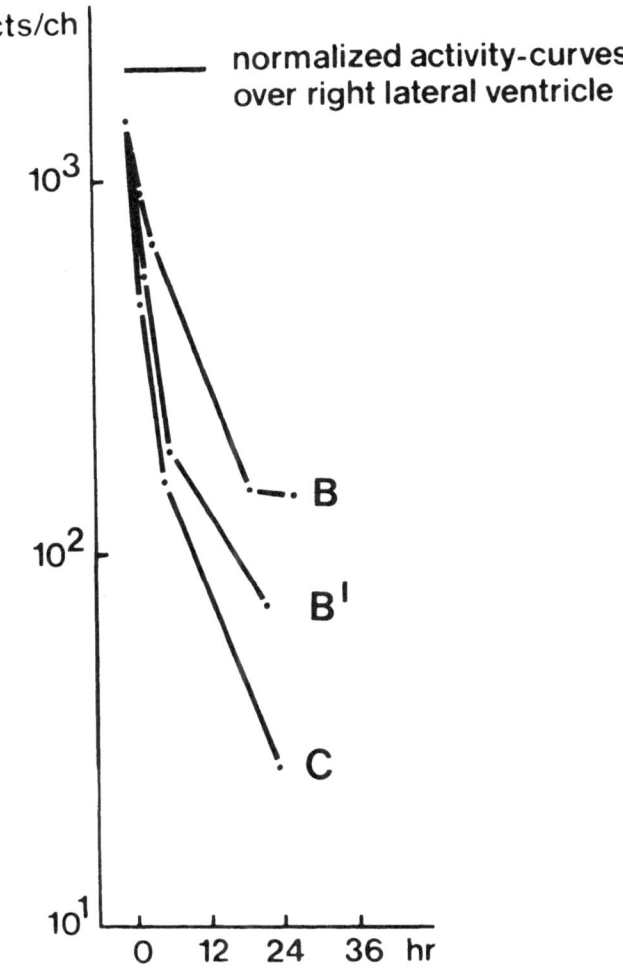

Fig. 6. Disappearance of 99m with normal Te-HSA from above the right ventricle measured in patient C (from figure 5)and patient B (from figure 7)) with abnormal circulation before (B) and improvement after treatment (B¹).

252

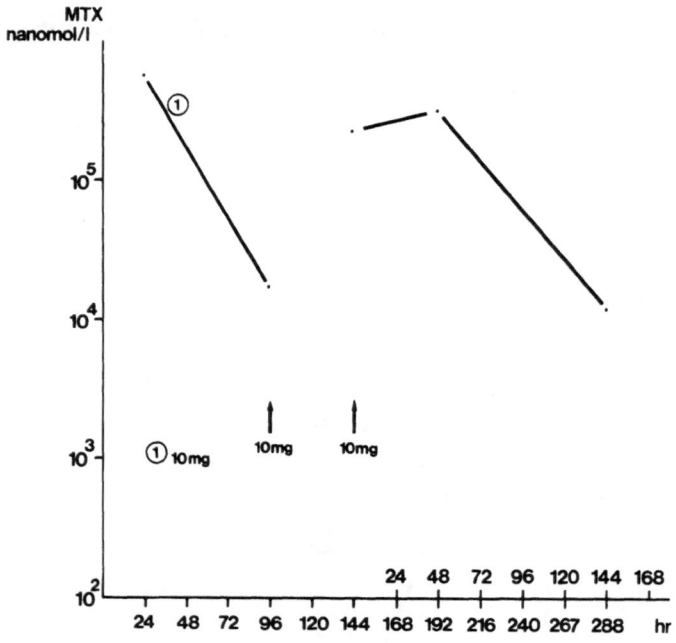

Fig. 7. MTX levels in CSF obtained by Ommaya reservoir puncture in patient B with meningeal extension of Non-Hodgkin lymphoma and diabetes insipidus. The disappearance of 29 hr Te-HSA is shown in figure 6 (patient B; B and B$^+$).

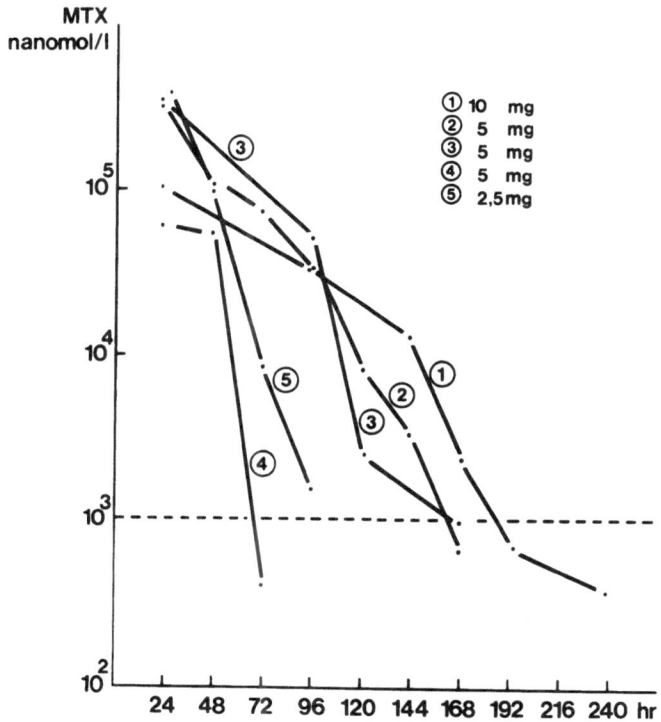

Fig. 8. MTX levels in CSF obtained by Ommaya reservoir puncture in a patient with breast cancer showing a more rapid disappearance after injection 4 and 5, parallel with improvement of clinical symptoms.

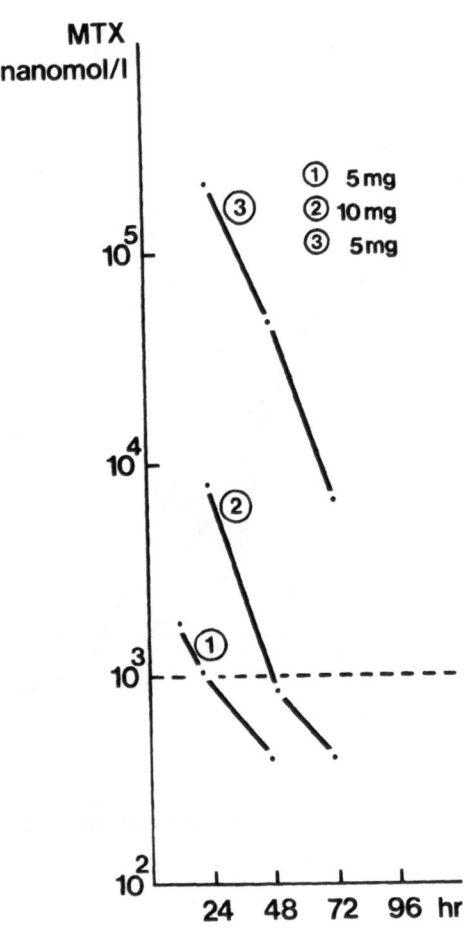

Fig. 9. MTX levels obtained by Ommaya reservoir puncture in a patient with breast cancer, and progression of CNS symptoms.

Toxicity intrathecal treatment

Acute
1. Arachnoiditis
2. Paresis
3. Encephalopathy

Chronic
1. Leukencephalopathy
2. Mineralizing angiopathy
3. C.T. scan abnormalities
4. Disturbances in intelligence and development

Table 2.

Factors influencing toxicity i.t. MTX

1. Solvents of MTX
2. Duration of exposition to MTX
   influenced by - dose given
                 - way of administration
                 - circulation CSF
                 - presence of disease
3. Combination with other treatments
                 - radiotherapy
                 - systemic drugs

Table 3.

Conclusions

The principles of treating meningeal leucaemia are generally agreed upon. In cases of meningeal lymphoma and solid meningeal metastases there is less experience. If the general condition of the patient and the prognosis of the primary disease are favourable treatment of meningeal metastases is worthwhile. C.T. brainscanning is important in excluding CNS metastases which make the prognosis poor. Administration of drugs to the CSF can be done best by use of an Ommaya system. Measurements of MTX levels in the CSF may be helpful to predict drug toxicity. Isotope ventriculography may be of value in indicating a delayed drug clearance. Remission following treatment of meningeal leucaemia occur in 90% with MTX administration, but maintenance treatment is necessary. In extensive localization of meningeal lymphoma and carcinomatosis possible in combination with intracerebral metastases intrathecal MTX administration is mostly combined with radiotherapy. In cases with meningeal lymphoma and carcinomatosis without gross impairment of the CSF circulation and without intracerebral localization remission induction with MTX only might be considered.

Acknowledgements

We should like to thank Dr. Persijn for the MTX determination in the CSF, Dr. Behrend for kindly giving the data of the MTX levels in children treated with high dose MTX, and Dr. Hoefnagel for the isotope studies.

References

Bleyer W.A., Pizzo P.A., Spence A.M., Platt W.D., Benjamin D.R., Kollins Ch.J., Poplack D.G.: The Ommaya Reservoir: Newly Recognized Complications and Recommendations for Insertion and Use. Cancer 41: 2431-2437, 1978.

Goedhart Z.D.: Het Ommaya Systeem, doctors thesis 1978, Leiden.

Jap H.W., Yap B.S. e.a.: Treatment and prognostic factors for meningeal carcinomatosis in breast cancer. Proceeding AACR and ASCO-meeting, 20/93, 1979.

Larson S.M., Johnston G.S., Ommaya A.K., Jones A.E., Di Chiro G.: The Radionuclide Ventriculogram. JAMA 224: 853-857, 1973.

McCullough D.C., Harbert J.C.: Isotope Demonstration of CSF Pathways. JAMA 209: 558-560, 1969.

Ommaya A.K.: Subcutaneous Reservoir and Pump for Sterile Access to Ventricular Cerebrospinal Fluid. The Lancet 2: 983-984, 1963.

Pochedly C.: Leukemia and lymphoma in the nervous system. Charles C. Thomas Publisher. Springfield, Illinois, U.S.A.

Shapiro W.R., Young D.F., Mehta B.M.: Metrotrexate: Distribution in Cerebrospinal Fluid after Intravenous, Ventricular and Lumbar Injections. The New England Journal of Medicine 293: 161-166, 1975.

Shapiro W.R., Posher J.B. e.a.: Treatment of Meningeal Neoplasms. Cancer Treatment Rep. 61: 733, 1977.

Waaij D. v.d.: Kolonisatie-resistentie van het Maagdarmkanaal; Nieuwe Wegen voor de Infectiepreventie in Ziekenhuis. Ned. T. v. Geneesk. 123: 273-276, 1979.

SHORT COMMUNICATIONS

22. THE ROLE WHICH VIRUSES MAY PLAY IN THE CAUSATION OF PARANEOPLASTIC NEUROLOGICAL SYNDROMES

H.E. Webb

Viruses may be involved in damaging the central nervous system in several different ways in association with neoplasia. Viral meningitis may occur as a result of immunosuppression produced by the disease process itself or by the drugs and irradiation used in therapy. (1,2) The actual virus involved in a particular case is seldom identified. Animal models such as Marek's disease (3), a herpes virus infection, in chickens causing lymphomas, polyneuritis and encephalitis have particular interest in relation to what may happen in human reticuloses and their associated neurological complications (4). Certain viruses of the Papova group which heavily infect the oligodendro-glia and cause focal demyelination in progressive multi-focal leucoencephalopathy (5) are tumour forming them-selves when inoculated into baby hamsters (6). Also, certain human tumours of the CNS have shown some evidence that the cells may have been infected with viruses and that this may have played some part in the tumour formation itself (7). The varied problems posed by the pathogenic potential of viruses in the CNS in relation to malignant diseases will be discussed with particular reference as to how our knowledge might be advanced further in this field.

REFERENCES

1. Webb, H. E. and Jagelman, S. In, Whitehouse, J. M. A. and Kay, H. E. M. (eds.), CNS Complications of Malignant Disease, The Macmillan Press Ltd., Basingstoke, Hampshire. 258-280, 1980.

2. Arnason, B. G. W. In, Rose, F. C. (ed.), Neuro-immunology, Blackwell Scientific Publications, Oxford. 1978.

3. Payne, L. N., Frazier, J. A. and Powell, P. C. In, Richter, G. W. and Epstein, M. A. (eds.), International Review of Experimental Pathology, Academi Press, New York.

4. Prineas, J. W. and Wright, R. G. Lab. Invest., 26, 548, 1972.

5. Mazlo, M. and Herndon, R. M. Neuropathology and Applied Neurobiology, 3, 323, 1977.

6. Walker, D. L., Padgett, B. L., ZuRhein, G. M., Albert, A. E. and Marsh, R. F. Science, (New York) 181, 674, 1973.

7. Weiss, A. F., Portmann, R., Fischer, H., Simm, J. and Zang, K. D. Proceed. Nat. Acad. Sci. (U.S.A.) 72, 609, 1975.

23. CFS-CYTOLOGY IN SECONDARY CNS MALIGNANCIES

G.Th.A.M. Bots

For already 80 years cytological examinations of the
Cerebro Spinal Fluid (C.S.F.) are performed to diagnose
diseases of the Central Nervous System (CNS). But it is
only in the last 15 years that marked improvements in the
technique of the preparation of the sediment established
it as a reliable diagnostic procedure. In Leyden, like in
most of Europe, we use the sedimentation chamber technique
introduced by Sayk about 20 years ago. This method is eco-
nomical, gives excellent conservation of the cells and for
one sediment only 1 ml fluid is necessary. May-Grünwald/
Giemsa is preferred by us as the staining of choice.

In normal CSF only a few monocytes and lymphocytes
are present. In many tumors the number of cells has increased, but this is largerly due to the accompanying inflammatory reaction or necrosis. Difficulties in the interpretat-
ion are increased when skin, bone marrow, cartilage, discus
or other elements are punctured and contaminate the sediment. Most metastases in the CNS are from carcinomas of the
bronchus, intestinal tract, mammary gland, or kidney, but
also melanoma, Hodgkin disease and non-Hodgkin lymphomas
are encountered. Very common is also arachnoidal involvement in acute lymphatic leukaemia.

Sometimes only a few tumorcells are present in the
CSF, but in the so-called carcinosis of the meninges an
overwhelming number of tumorcells is present. Often however
no cytological changes are observed because there is no
free communication between the metastasis and the CSF space
or so few cells are exfoliated from the tumor that they are
not present in every sample that is investigated by us.

A false-positive diagnosis of metastatic tumor may
a.o. occur in:
1. Colloid cyst of the 3rd ventricle, craniopharyngeoma,
epidermoid cyst, dermoid cyst, pituitary adenoma, ependy-

moma, plexus papilloma, undifferentiated glioma and other
primary intracranial tumor.
2. In hydrocephalus when atypical ependymal cells are
present.
3. Proliferation of arachnoidal cells and of macrophages.

False-negative results may occur when:
1. Not enough CSF is available for cytological investigation.
2. There is no access of the tumorcells to the CSF compartment that can be drained by the puncture.

A number of slides of metastatic tumorcells and of
carcinosis are presented.

So far we investigated the CSF in 60 patients with
cerebral metastasis. In 20% of them tumorcells were present
in the CSF. In these cases on an average only 1½ ml fluid
was used for sedimentation, so that very probably these
results could be improved by investigation of more fluid.
These results are better than those of the 270 cases of
primary CNS tumors we investigated. Than in only 15% of
them we detected praeoperatively tumorcells in the CSF. In
these cases on an average 2½ ml of CSF was investigated. In
cases of carcinosis of the meninges in 100% of the 12 cases
tumorcells could be detected in the CSF.

REFERENCES
1. Balhuizen, J.C., Bots, G.Th.A.M., Schaberg, A. and
   Bosman, F.T., Value of cerebrospinal fluid cytology for
   the diagnosis of malignancies in the central nervous
   system. J. Neurosurg. 48:747-753, 1978
2. Kölmel, H.W., Atlas of cerebrospinal fluid cells.
   Springer Verlag Berlin, Heidelberg, New York, 1976.
3. Oehmichen, M., Cerebrospinal fluid cytology. George
   Thieme Verlag Stuttgart, 1976
4. Sayk, J., Cytologie der Cerebrospinalflüssigkeit.
   Gustav Fischer Jena, 1960.
5. Schmidt, R.M., Cytological atlas of cerebrospinal fluid.
   Johann Ambrosius Barth Leipzig, 1978